CREW RESOURCE MANAGEMENT:

The flight plan for lasting change in patient safety

F. Andrew (Drew) Gaffney MD, FACC
Captain Stephen W. Harden
Rhea Seddon, MD

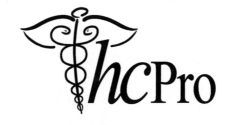

F. Andrew Gaffney, MD, FACC, Co-author

Captain Stephen W. Harden

Rhea Seddon, MD

Janet Spiegel, Managing Editor

Paul Amos, Group Publisher

Mike Mirabello, Senior Graphic Artist

Jackie Diehl Singer, Layout Artist

Pat Campagnone, Cover Designer

Jean St. Pierre, Director of Operations

Advice given is general. Readers should consult professional counsel for specific legal, ethical, or clinical questions. Arrangements can be made for quantity discounts. For more information, contact:

HCPro, Inc.
P.O. Box 1168
Marblehead, MA 01945
Telephone: 800/650-6787 or 781/639-1872
Fax: 781/639-2982
E-mail: *customerservice@hcpro.com*

Visit HCPro at its World Wide Web sites: *www.hcpro.com* and *www.hcmarketplace.com*

Rev. 08/2007
21256

CONTENTS

ABOUT THE AUTHORS

F. Andrew (Drew) Gaffney MD, FACC

F. Andrew (Drew) Gaffney MD, FACC, is professor of medical education and administration; professor of medicine; and attending physician at Vanderbilt University Medical Center in Nashville, TN. Gaffney is also the associate dean for clinical affairs and chief quality and patient safety officer at Vanderbilt University Medical Center.

Born and raised in New Mexico, he received his undergraduate degree from University of California–Berkeley and his MD from the University of New Mexico in Albuquerque. After completing his internal medicine training at Metro General Hospital in Cleveland and a cardiology fellowship at University of Texas Southwestern in Dallas, he remained on the faculty as a cardiologist.

From 1984–1991, he was assigned to the Johnson Space Center in Houston as a payload specialist and flew aboard the space shuttle Columbia June 5–14, 1991. This flight, Spacelab Life Sciences 1, was a highly successful science mission examining physiological adaptation to microgravity. He received the National Spaceflight Medal, a National Aeronautics and Space Administration (NASA) Group Achievement Award and, along with a crewmate, the first Flight Surgeon-Astronaut wings ever granted by the United States Air Force. He continues to serve in the Air Force Reserve as a researcher and senior flight-surgeon astronaut. Gaffney is also a commercial pilot with ratings in both airplanes and gliders.

In 1992, he joined the Vanderbilt faculty as chief of clinical cardiology. He maintains an active cardiology practice at Vanderbilt and is listed in "America's Best Doctors."

In 2001, Gaffney spent a year at Sweden's Karolinska Institutet and founded its Center for Patient Safety. He is currently an adjunct professor there and continues to do patient safety and medical malpractice prevention research.

Gaffney's work in patient safety and crew resource management (CRM) is a natural extension of his experience in medicine, aerospace, and organizational change. He has coauthored more than 100 scientific papers and holds eight patents. His goal is to help make Vanderbilt America's safest hospital using aviation-based safety tools.

Captain Stephen W. Harden

Captain Stephen W. Harden is president of LifeWings Partners, LLC, and cofounder of Crew Training International, Inc. (CTI), the parent company of LifeWings. Harden has been the principal architect of LifeWing's adaptation of aviation-based safety tools and practices for healthcare. In 2005, he was responsible for the CRM courseware and training provided to more than 12,000 physicians and staff.

Prior to assuming his position at LifeWings, Harden was the principal courseware designer of CTI's CRM training for the U.S. Air Combat Command, Air National Guard, Air Force Reserve Command, Italian Air Force, Swiss Air Force, Belgian Air Force, domestic and commercial airlines, construction crews, and hospital surgical teams. He has overseen the production of more than 40 separate courses for a wide variety of military and commercial customers. He has also served on the instructional staff of the University of Southern California's School of Aviation Safety.

While managing the CTI Courseware Development Division, Harden also served as senior course developer for all CRM training programs for Federal Express. At FedEx, he designed, developed, and delivered more than 12 comprehensive training courses encompassing more than 90 hours of instruction. His expertise in the field of courseware development has garnered him four personal "Bravo Zulu" awards for superior performance and one organizational award for quality achievement. Harden was recognized in 1993 by FedEx senior management as the individual who had contributed the most to the safety of FedEx flight operations.

Harden is a graduate of the United States Naval Academy. He accumulated more than 300 aircraft carrier landings during his service with the Navy and was selected to be an instructor pilot at the Navy's elite Fighter Weapons School (TOPGUN). He holds an Airline Transport Pilot rating and Type ratings in B-727 and 737 aircraft and is an Federal Aviation Administration–certified flight examiner.

Rhea Seddon, MD

Rhea Seddon, MD, is the assistant chief medical officer of the Vanderbilt Medical Group in Nashville, TN, and an assistant professor of medical administration and education at Vanderbilt University Medical Center. She currently coleads an initiative aimed at improving patient safety and quality of care by the use of an aviation-based model of CRM. She is a member of the Executive Safety Committee and the Faculty Training Committee. She has been involved in a variety of quality improvement efforts for the medical center.

Prior to coming to Vanderbilt, Seddon spent 19 years with NASA. In 1978 she was selected as one of the first six women to enter the astronaut program. She flew aboard her first Shuttle flight in 1985, deployed two satellites, operated the Remote Manipulator Arm, and performed the first echocardiography in space. She was selected to serve as a mission specialist on the first shuttle flight dedicated entirely to life sciences research, Spacelab Life Sciences 1, in 1991. In 1993, Seddon was the payload commander in charge of all science activities on Spacelab Life Sciences 2 and performed the first animal dissections in space. This brought her total time in space to 30 days.

While at NASA Seddon served in many roles, including flying as a rescue helicopter physician for the first shuttle flights and helping to develop the Shuttle Medical Kit and the checklist for space medical operations. She was also involved in crew recovery operations following the Challenger accident. Seddon was a member of NASA's Institutional Review Board and the International Bioethics Task Force. After leaving NASA, she was appointed to numerous space advisory committees including two Institute of Medicine committees looking at astronaut health, and is on the Board of Trust of Universities Space Research Association.

A graduate of the University of California at Berkeley with a degree in physiology, Seddon received her MD degree from the University of Tennessee College of Medicine in Memphis where she completed her residency in general surgery. She has performed research on the effects of nutrition in cancer patients undergoing radiation therapy and served as an emergency physician part-time during her residency and her years at NASA.

ACKNOWLEDGEMENTS

The authors wish to acknowledge and thank their colleagues and coworkers Jeffrey Hill of Vanderbilt University and Richard Clark and Michael Osborn of Lifewings Partners, LLC, for their insights and suggestions while applying crew resource management to healthcare. The authors are also grateful to Rodney Williams and James Bagian of the U.S Department of Veterans' Affairs National Center for Patient Safety and Johan Thor of the Karolinska Institutet in Stockholm, Sweden for their review and thoughtful suggestions.

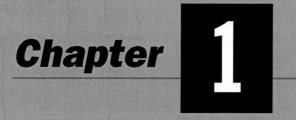

Chapter 1

UNDERSTANDING THE CONCEPT OF CREW RESOURCE MANAGEMENT AND HOW IT CAN HELP HEALTHCARE

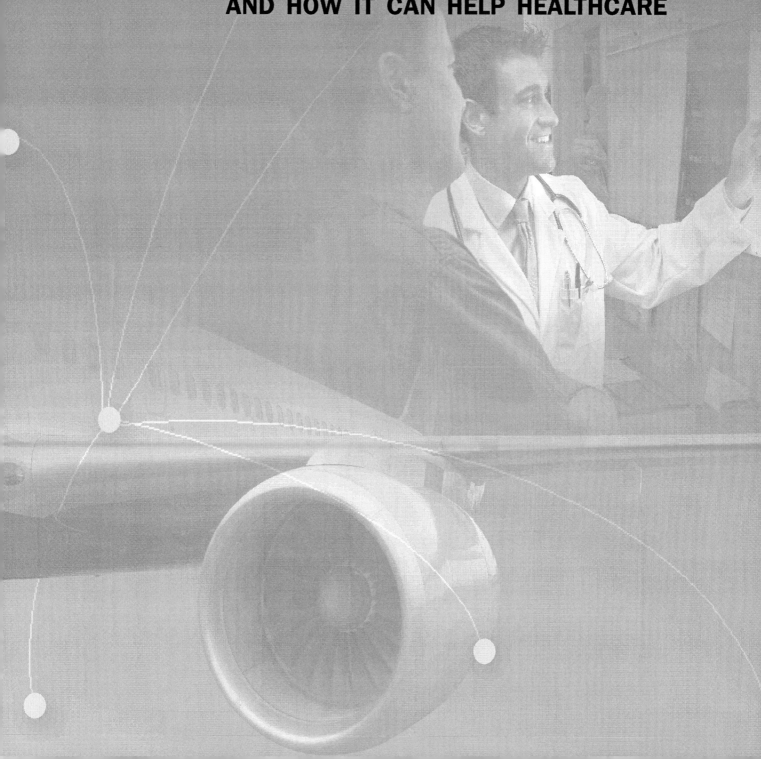

Chapter 1

UNDERSTANDING THE CONCEPT OF CREW RESOURCE MANAGEMENT AND HOW IT CAN HELP HEALTHCARE

What is crew resource management and why did aviation pursue it?

Fireballs, mangled metal, passengers dying hundreds at a time, and grim newspaper headlines led aviation on a path to crew resource management (CRM). Understanding the concept of CRM as a safety system begins with understanding the history of aviation mishaps. The dismal record of modern air disasters sheds light on the birth of CRM. Aviation's worst disaster ever, a collision between two jumbo jets, provided the strongest catalyst for airlines to develop a "different way of doing things" that ultimately became CRM.

On March 27, 1977, Captain Jacob Van Zanten expertly guided his B-747 jumbo jet onto the fog-shrouded runway on Tenerife Island in the Azores. Stern experienced and knowledgeable—he was the senior B-747 instructor pilot for his airline. His copilot for that flight had received his training to operate the B-747 from Captain Van Zanten just six months earlier.

Despite his 30-plus years of experience, Captain Van Zanten was about to make a fatal error: he began his takeoff roll without clearance from the control tower. Neither his copilot nor his flight engineer were certain whether a takeoff clearance had been received, and both strongly suspected that another airplane was on the runway hidden in the fog. Both made weak hints to their captain, seemingly reluctant to offend or anger him. The captain brusquely dismissed both hints and shoved the throttles forward bringing to life hundreds of thousands of pounds of thrust and accelerated the jet toward destruction.

Moments later, its speed increasing rapidly, the 747 emerged from the fog. In that awful moment, Captain Van Zanten most assuredly realized his error as his windscreen filled with a horrible sight—another 747 blocking his path on the runway. In that instant, the aircraft commander realized he was moving too quickly to stop before smashing into the other airplane and too slowly to get airborne and fly over it. Death for him, his crew, and all his passengers was just seconds away.

In the other airplane, the copilot was the first to see the onrushing jet. He began to scream to his captain, "Get off! Get Off! Get Off!" as he shoved the throttles forward in a desperate attempt to taxi off the runway and onto the grass. He was too late. Moments later, the airplanes collided in a thunderous fireball. The resulting fire consumed 583 lives, making it the worst disaster in aviation history.

The resulting accident investigation (similar to a root-cause analysis in healthcare) revealed a tragic chain of events rooted in human error. Poor communication, flawed teamwork, rushed procedures, and time pressure all contributed to the deadly outcome.

Unfortunately this was only the first in a long series of tragic aviation accidents, all with a similar root cause—human error. Some of these disasters include the following:

- A United Airlines DC-8 crashed in Portland, OR, when a very senior and experienced captain, while troubleshooting a malfunctioning landing gear and after failing to heed the veiled warnings of his crew, ran out of fuel and crash-landed in the trees just short of the runway.

- An Air Florida B-737 crashed into the Potomac River at Washington (DC) National Airport when two experienced pilots miscommunicated about the proper engine settings during a snowstorm.

- A USAir B-737 slid into the river at New York's La Guardia airport when an experienced captain failed to realize his copilot was on his first trip after completion of training. He allowed the copilot to attempt a take-off in wet, slick conditions. The inexperienced copilot made a mistake from which the captain could not recover, leading to tragic consequences.

These are just four accidents in a long list of similar mishaps that led NASA to publish research showing that **70%–80% of all aviation accidents were caused by human error in a team setting** and that pilot error was more likely to reflect failures in team communication and coordination than deficiencies in technical proficiency.[1]

At first, aviation's reaction to the increasing accident rate was to try to harness the power of the computer and new technology (much the same way some healthcare organizations have attempted to do so). Airplanes were literally stuffed with "black boxes" designed to prevent accidents. But after a series of technology-related accidents, including the loss of a brand new airplane, an Airbus A-320, the aviation industry realized technology alone was not the answer. In that accident, the pilots tried to demonstrate the ability of the computer-assisted flight controls to rescue the airplane from a stall, but instead caused a crash. The Airbus pilots waited for the computer to take over the flight controls. When it didn't respond as they thought it would, and under the stress of the moment, the pilots pushed the wrong buttons in the cockpit. The airplane flew into the trees at the end of the runway.

The eye-opening conclusion was that no matter how advanced the technological system, **if humans are involved, error is inevitable.** This Airbus accident demonstrated that new technology may reduce risk of error, but it can also introduce new opportunity for error. The lesson learned was that technology can help, but it is not the complete answer.

This conclusion—that error is inevitable when human beings are involved—became the key to reducing the air accident rate. Aviation trainers and system designers accepted the fact that human beings are not perfect and never will be. Although we have more knowledge and technology is better, the human brain, which processes the knowledge and uses the technology, is unchanged. Physiological and psychological properties of our brain make us prone to errors.

The key to better safety and fewer accidents is managing the inevitable error

Aviation and other high-reliability organizations now manage (as healthcare is beginning to) these inevitable errors by doing two things:

1. Training teams to use specific teamwork and communication behaviors.

2. Implementing safety tools (e.g., procedures, protocols, checklists, etc.) that complement those behaviors to detect and trap small errors before they become serious or even fatal mistakes.

CRM, whether used in aviation or healthcare, is a combination of teamwork and communication behaviors, and the safety tools that support those behaviors.

Teamwork skills and safety tools are a powerful combination that provides error-stopping results

FIGURE 1.1

Teamwork skills + **Safety tools**

A real-life example of CRM in action occurs every day when a cockpit crew is given a clearance by Air Traffic Control (ATC) to climb to a new altitude. The flight crew will acknowledge the new instructions from ATC and "read back" the exact altitude to which the flight has been cleared. ATC will listen for this read back and, if it is not received, will query the crew as to whether they heard the instruction. Should the crew read back an altitude different from the one given, ATC can immediately intervene and correct the mistake. This cross-check prevents collisions between aircraft. Both parts of the CRM safety system are seen here: precise communication between flight crews and ATC (communication skill) and the standard operating procedure of providing a read back (safety tool).

The results of using CRM in aviation

As the CRM system became widespread in aviation, dramatic decreases in accident rates occurred in a variety of related organizations that used CRM as well. For example,

- military transport squadrons reduced accidents by 52%[2]

- Navy aircraft reduced accidents by 81%[3]

- helicopter accidents declined by 54%[4]

- major U.S. airlines, at the time this book was published, had no passenger fatalities since the fall of 2001—almost four years[5]

CRM was so effective that it became required by all aviation organizations. In 1992, the Federal Aviation Administration (FAA) required CRM programs to be established at all U.S. airlines. The military and other government flight organizations quickly followed suit. Not long afterward, foreign airlines and military flight units also required CRM in their operations.

CRM-like systems are used in many other high-risk industries. Nuclear-powered submarines, nuclear power and chemical manufacturing plants, and seaborne commercial shipping lines all use safety systems that include teamwork training and specific safety tools such as checklists and standard procedures. In fact, all modern high-reliability organizations use some form of CRM to manage human fallibility and achieve safety in otherwise potentially dangerous environments. Healthcare, with a growing awareness of its own statistics on errors and patient injuries, is beginning to take notice of the results achieved by aviation and its CRM program.

Why is CRM needed in healthcare?

CRM is consistent with the principle of "first, do no harm." This is the core tenet in healthcare and both a personal and an institutional obligation. Healthcare leaders must encourage, support, and sponsor programs that make patient safety the absolute prerequisite and cornerstone of quality care. Organizations and their employees must assure patients that they will be safe from medical errors and accidents.

Healthcare workers at all levels are professionally and personally committed and work hard to provide the best possible care to their patients, but medical errors and mishaps continue to occur at unacceptably high rates. "Working harder" or "paying closer attention" will not prevent the majority of medical errors—new tools and skills are clearly needed, and CRM can provide them.

CRM provides a 'safe practice dividend'

Errors cost money. The impact to the organization's bottom line in malpractice costs and loss of productive time due to a major error can ruin the best of hospitals. Prestige and reputation suffer. Bad publicity erodes market share. Employee morale sinks. Productivity evaporates. Almost all healthcare workers have been involved in a patient-injuring error and have experienced the guilt, shame, and sadness that can sometimes last a lifetime. The Institute of Medicine (IOM) estimates the annual cost of errors in U.S. hospitals to be approximately $17 billion each year. A Danish government-sponsored study showed that approximately one-seventh of all hospital days resulted from preventable medical errors. For every error a CRM program detects and corrects before it hurts a patient, dollars are saved. How much improvement could be made in healthcare, and how many more people could obtain needed care with even a portion of this "safe practice dividend"?

CRM in complex systems provides an error rate significantly better than those in healthcare

Figure 1.2 shows a graph of error rates across a variety of systems and groups them according to their rates of error per "operation," ranging from dangerous to ultrasafe. Notice where hospitals fall.

Most patients and healthcare workers would find it disturbing to know that a hospital stay has the same degree of danger as bungee jumping or motorcycle racing.

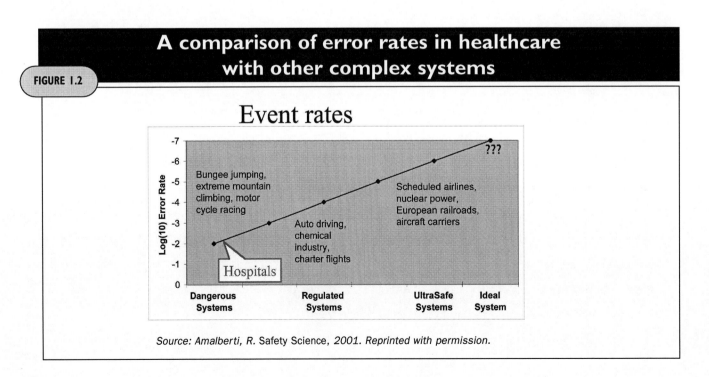

FIGURE 1.2

A comparison of error rates in healthcare with other complex systems

Source: Amalberti, R. Safety Science, 2001. Reprinted with permission.

Another study by Robert Galvin, MD, the Director of Global Healthcare for General Electric, looked at defects per million operations (DPMO) in aviation and hospital care. Scheduled major airlines have greatly exceeded the coveted "Six Sigma" (a measure of nearly perfect reliability) in safe operations. However, no healthcare process approaches this level of safety. According to this study, a patient is more likely to get his baggage delivered at his destination than he is to receive the right medication as an inpatient. See Figure 1.3 for statistics on Defects Per Million Opportunities (DPMO).

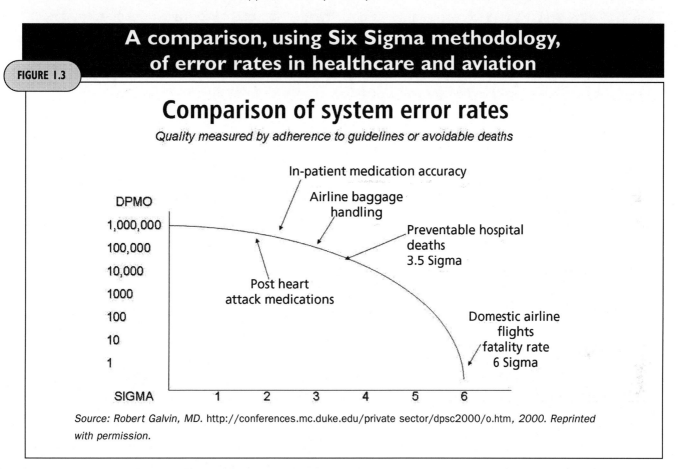

FIGURE 1.3

A comparison, using Six Sigma methodology, of error rates in healthcare and aviation

Comparison of system error rates

Quality measured by adherence to guidelines or avoidable deaths

Source: Robert Galvin, MD. http://conferences.mc.duke.edu/private sector/dpsc2000/o.htm, 2000. Reprinted with permission.

In general, patients aren't aware of the healthcare system's poor record. The much-publicized 1999 IOM report, To Err Is Human, estimated that between 44,000 and 98,000 deaths per year occur in U.S. hospitals due to preventable error. In its recommendations to address this problem, the IOM suggested CRM as one solution for this serious national patient safety problem.

CRM is strongly recommended by leading healthcare organizations

The Joint Commission on Accreditation of Healthcare Organizations (JCAHO), the IOM, the Accreditation

Council for Graduate Medical Education (ACGME), and others recognize the usefulness of CRM training and safety tools. The JCAHO requires hospitals to adopt some of the proven safety tools from ultrasafe organizations. In 2003 the JCAHO required that a time out be conducted prior to procedures to eliminate wrong surgeries. The time out is similar to the preflight briefing done by all flight crews before each takeoff.

In 2005, the JCAHO required "read back" of verbal orders and other important healthcare information, and in 2006, it requires hospitals to develop a standardized "handoff" of patient information when patient care is transferred from one caregiver to another. This is a concept and model adopted from aviation. For example, when switching from one ATC center to another, pilots and controllers follow a specific protocol designed to prevent errors and ensure precise, continuous control of aircraft.

The ACGME has also adopted some of the basic concepts of CRM by making communication, system-based practice, and continuous improvement core competencies that residents must master during their training. Along with medical knowledge and technical training, young physicians learn that they must communicate, make good decisions, and function as part of a team to reach their highest potential.

The IOM identified six dimensions of the ideal healthcare system. It must be safe, effective, patient-centered, timely, efficient, and equitable. It was perhaps no accident that "safe" was listed as the first aim that must be achieved. Without safety, the other dimensions become irrelevant. To achieve patient safety, a coordinated program such as CRM must be put in place.

CRM programs help hospitals achieve Leapfrog certification

Wanting their employees and family members to use only those hospitals with the best level of safety and quality, purchasers of healthcare services are evaluating the hospitals where they send patients. The Leapfrog Group, an initiative driven by organizations that buy healthcare and work to initiate breakthrough improvements in the safety, quality, and affordability of healthcare for Americans, has specified criteria by which facilities can be rated according to recognized standards. Over 25% of points in the group's current scoring system relate to a "culture of safety." Patient safety practices gaining points under this rating system include team training, checklists, read back of information, handoffs, and verification—all components of CRM.

CRM programs help protect a hospital's reputation with the public

Best-selling books like Internal Bleeding and Complications tell compelling stories from physicians' first-hand experience of how serious errors can occur. A May 2005 article in Oprah Winfrey's magazine, O, titled, "When bad medicine happens to good people" also reached a large audience. Additionally, the public is beginning to demand information about their healthcare providers. Healthcare rating Web sites, such as the Centers for Medicare & Medicaid Services' www.hospitalcompare.hhs.gov, are increasingly available. Both physicians and hospitals are now being profiled on everything from error rates to bedside manner. Significant, headline-making errors become widely known through a variety of media and affect public perception of a facility's quality. CRM programs can provide a competitive advantage in the marketplace because hospitals can make their communities aware that they use proven methods to ensure safety and quality.

CRM programs add to the bottom line

The business case for CRM programs is compelling. Institutions creating better leaders, teams, coordination, and communication become the employers of choice and recoup the significant costs of high staff and physician turnover. Some malpractice insurance companies now offer rebates to physicians who attend courses in teamwork and communication to learn how to prevent error. Self-insured institutions are considering cuts in departmental premiums for behavior change toward safety. Institutions recognize that the cost of errors and high turnover come straight from the bottom line. A change in attitude is occurring: Payouts for medical errors are not just the "cost of doing business," but rather an expense that can be managed and reduced by improving patient safety.

Has CRM worked in healthcare?

Hospital executives with profit and loss responsibility want to know whether CRM works. Effectively implemented CRM programs do work in healthcare and produce results. CRM results appearing in peer-reviewed journals and other publications include

- a 50% reduction in surgical counts errors[6]
- clinical error rate reductions from 30% to 4.4%[7]
- a 53% reduction in adverse outcomes[8]
- a 55% reduction in observed errors[9]
- teamwork and communication skills, more than previous surgical experience, determine how quickly medical personnel develop expertise with new technology (e.g, robotics for minimally invasive cardiac surgery)[10]

Healthcare institutions that have implemented CRM programs have observed

- a 10-fold reduction in wrong surgeries
- an improvement in pre-procedure antibiotic administration from 68% to 96%
- a 30% reduction in nurse turnover
- a statistically significant improvement in employee satisfaction survey responses

In our own institution, Vanderbilt University Medical Center in Nashville, TN, there have been changes in caregivers' attitudes, behavior, and outcomes after CRM training and implementation. An article by Grogan et al. in the December 2004 Journal of the American College of Surgeons shows a significant shift in the attitudes of our staff toward safety and an increase in teamwork after training in CRM skills. Vanderbilt has implemented safety tools in the cath lab and operating room (OR) to support the teamwork behaviors learned during the training. Direct observation of behavior shows that almost all procedures in those departments are now preceded by a prebrief. Cath lab personnel report greater efficiency and safety. Our employee satisfaction survey results show greater satisfaction among Vanderbilt's employees who have received CRM training and work in departments that have implemented CRM safety tools.

The implementation of CRM in all high-reliability organizations has dramatically reduced accident rates and saved thousands of lives and billions of dollars for those organizations. Perhaps because of these savings, no high-reliability organization has chosen to perform a randomized, placebo-controlled trial of CRM. The absence of such trials is often used as an argument against the adoption of CRM by healthcare. The authors understand this concern but believe there are compelling arguments for proceeding with widespread CRM implementation. Here are a few reasons for proceeding with CRM now:

- There is no alternative therapy (i.e., there are currently no "safe" hospitals in America).

- CRM is a well-established, well-understood program that has been applied to a variety of disparate, complex, high-risk industries with comparable success in all.

- The risk-benefit ratio for CRM is greatly in favor of benefit. The only risk to CRM is cost, and that's trivial compared to overall healthcare expenditures resulting from medical errors.

- To date, full implementation of CRM has not been accomplished in any U.S. hospital. If results in healthcare are anywhere close to what's been seen in other industries, comparison with "historical controls" will provide strong support for CRM's effectiveness in healthcare.

- Careful measurement of CRM outcomes, as described in this book, should be performed in any CRM implementation. This will produce data which can be used to drive the decision as to whether to proceed with CRM implementation in healthcare.

Ultimately, no matter how logical and convincing the data concerning improvements made by CRM programs are, nothing convinces others about the usefulness of CRM as much as the individual stories of harm and injury averted by the culture of safety created by CRM. These stories create enthusiasm and passion for CRM and its contribution to the mission of saving and healing lives.

Case study on CRM success

Here is a case study based on a true story that demonstrates how a successfully implemented CRM program changes behavior and allows the caregiving team to detect and correct errors before they harm the patient.

Two patients, Mr. Romero and Mr. Reynaldo, were scheduled for surgery on the same day. Because he arrived late and due to misunderstanding in admitting, Mr. Romero was misidentified and received Mr. Reynaldo's armband. No one noticed that he was hard of hearing. Although he wore a hearing aid, he relied mostly on lip reading.

In the preoperative holding room, the nurse asked, "Are you Mr. Reynaldo?"

"Yes," said Mr. Romero, since the two names were similar.

The nurse took the papers he brought from admitting (also under the name Reynaldo) and pulled up the electronic medical record under this name. She showed these to the certified registered nurse anesthetist (CRNA) who came to see the patient. The CRNA saw that a good history and physical was on the chart, the preoperative orders were written, and the operative permit was signed. She asked the patient the usual questions about any interim illness, when he had last eaten, and so on and then did a brief physical exam. Everything seemed to be in order.

The surgery resident then stopped by to see the patient. Because of the 80-hour work rule, he had not seen this patient previously. He introduced himself to the patient and checked the armband and the chart.

"Can you tell me what procedure you're supposed to have done today," the resident asked as he prepared to mark the patient's arm for creation of an arterio-venous fistula, as listed in the consent form (for Mr. Reynaldo).

The patient looked at him and said, "I am here to have my aorta done."

The resident rechecked the armband and the operative permit. Was this elderly man confused? Having attended CRM class, the resident thought for a moment and remembered that he had learned that the patient was part of his team and that patients often provide important cross-checking information. The ambiguity between the chart and the patient's response was clearly a red flag. The resident also remembered the maxim "See it, say it, fix it!" and asked the patient to state his full name.

"Oscar Roberto Romero" he replied.

Had the question not been asked, the patient probably would not have questioned the marks on his arm. The patient would perhaps have been taken to the OR, sedated, prepped, and draped. The attending surgeon might have arrived just in time to help the resident with the case. Imagine Mr. Romero's surprise when he awoke with an unneeded fistula in his arm and an untreated abdominal aortic obstruction.

More important, who had gotten Mr. Romero's armband? Of course, it was Mr. Reynaldo, who spoke no English. He had brought a young granddaughter who barely spoke English herself to translate. She was too shy to question the "mispronunciation" of her grandfather's name, and she was not familiar with his medical problems or the planned procedure for dialysis for his chronic renal failure. What could have been the outcome if the patient had been hustled through the system and an aortic Y-graft had been performed, despite his poor medical condition?

This story and the hundred others like it make a truly compelling case for adoption of CRM in healthcare. Two near misses were recognized, and one potential death was avoided. The right care to the right patient at the right time occurred because of a system that provides teamwork training and safety tools to detect and correct the inevitable human errors that occur when providing care in a complex environment.

End notes

1. G. E. Cooper, M. D. White and J. K. Lauber, Eds., *Resource management on the flightdeck: Proceedings of a NASA/Industry workshop*, (NASA CP-2120, Moffett Field, CA, NASA-Ames Research Center, 1980).

2. Alan Diehl, *Does Cockpit Management Training Reduce Aircrew Error?* Paper presented during the 22nd International Seminar International Society of Air Safety Investigators, Canberra, Australia, November 1991.

3. Ibid.

4. Ibid.

5. "Fatal Airliner Events," AirSafe.Com, *www.airsafe.com/events/fatal01.htm* (accessed July 17, 2005).

6. R. M. Rivers, Diane Swain and Bill Nixon, "Using aviation safety measures to enhance patient outcomes," *AORN Journal* 2003; 77:158.

7. J. C. Morey and others, "Error Reduction and Performance Improvement in the Emergency Department through Formal Teamwork Training: Evaluation results of the MedTeams project," *Health Service Results* 2002; 37:1553.

8. Marion Garza and J. S. Piver, "Can Aviation Safety Methods Cut Obstetric Errors?" *OB/GYN Malpractice Prevention* 11, No. 8 (August 2004): 57–64.

9. "Beyond Blame: Ob-Gyns Investigating Model Reforms On Patient Safety," ACOG News Release, *www.acog.org/from_home/publications/press_releases/nr05-03-04.cfm* (accessed July 17, 2005).

10. G. P. Pisano and others, "Organizational difference in rates of learning: Evidence from the adoption of minimally invasive cardiac surgery," *Management Science* 47, No. 6 (June 2001): 752.

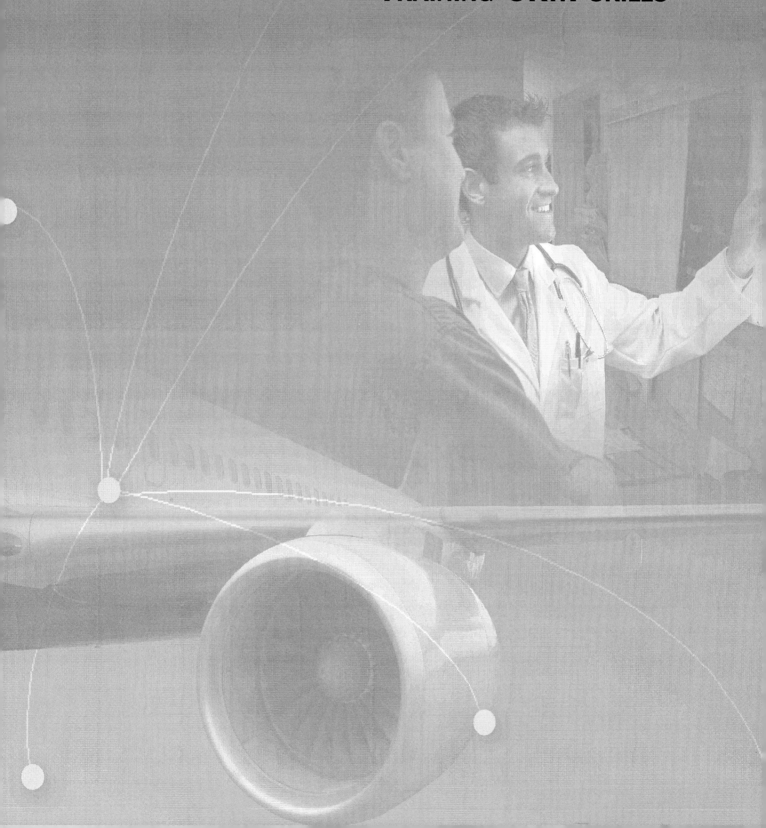

Chapter 2

TRAINING CRM SKILLS

Chapter 2

TRAINING CRM SKILLS

A computer needs both software and hardware to work correctly. Software without hardware is useless. Hardware without software to bring it alive is also worthless. Effective CRM systems have a similar problem: They need both software and hardware to work effectively. Think of CRM's software as the behaviors that result from the teamwork and communications training, and the hardware as the safety tools that require and support the use of the behaviors.

For example, checking the patient's armband against the medical record and conducting this check in conjunction with another caregiver is an example of teamwork behavior. Implementing a **time-out** briefing as a standard operating procedure and including the check of the patient's ID during that briefing is an example of a safety tool that supports and requires the teamwork behavior.

Thus we have software (i.e., the cross-checking teamwork behaviors) and hardware (i.e., the required **time-out** briefing being conducted with a written checklist) working together to create an effective CRM system.

An important point for organizations considering the implementation of a CRM program is that training (i.e., skills-based seminars) without the implementation of aviation-based safety tools will not produce the patient safety results you seek.

Train staff in teamwork and communication

Effective CRM training programs equip staff with two individual skills (i.e., behaviors that can be used independently or as part of a team). These are the

1) skills needed as countermeasures to combat the effects of fatigue.

2) ability to recognize the warning signs that an error chain is building and might result in an adverse event or outcome. These warning signs are commonly called **red flags.**

Equipped with these skills, personnel must then learn how to

- rapidly and effectively build a team from people with diverse personalities and technical talents

- communicate effectively with precision and without regard to rank or position when safety is at risk

- recognize **red flags** and communicate to the team what they mean

- recognize and mitigate the effects of fatigue on performance and cross-check and back up their actions

- use effective team problem-solving and decision-making skills when time and circumstances permit

- provide performance feedback to one another in a specific and nonthreatening way that promotes learning and improves performance for the next time

Each CRM skill builds on the others (Figure 2.1 and Table 2.1) with the ultimate goal of making the best decisions for patient safety. The degree to which team leaders and followers can create a team will determine how effectively information will flow between the members of the team. The ability of the team to communicate effectively and precisely will determine the quality of their responses when **red flags** are noted or the effects of fatigue are present. Additionally, the quality of the team building and communication

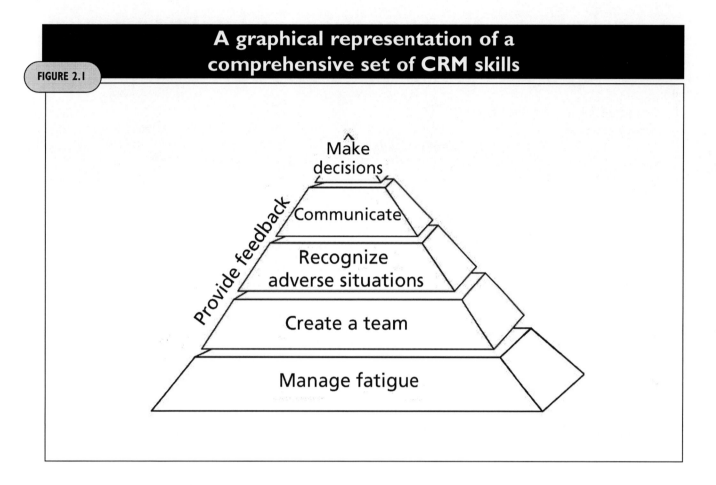

FIGURE 2.1

A graphical representation of a comprehensive set of CRM skills

Make decisions

Communicate

Recognize adverse situations

Create a team

Manage fatigue

Provide feedback

flow will determine the team's ability to avoid common decision-making errors. Finally, no learning will occur during performance feedback without a sense of team and open communication flow.

Be forewarned: The inclusion of fatigue countermeasures as part of a training curriculum for a medical audience will meet resistance. Many in healthcare see fatigue as a constant companion of their profession and an expected byproduct of providing 24/7 service. Yet the effects of fatigue are severe and do cause errors that harm patients.[1] One study estimates that 24 hours of wakefulness has the same effect on attention span, reaction time, and memory as having a Blood Alcohol Content of 0.10.[2] Driving in this condition will justify arrest in most states, yet many healthcare organizations think nothing of providing patient care with staff at this level of fatigue. Exhaustion and fatigue are indeed constant companions of the healthcare provider, just as they are of the pilot flying a week of all-night "red-eye specials," or the nuclear power plant operator on his fourth consecutive midnight shift.

	Learning objectives for a comprehensive CRM skills training course
TABLE 2.1	

Introduction to aviation-based CRM safety programs
- State the effect of CRM on aviation accident and incident rates
- Understand the similarities between healthcare and aviation
- Discuss recent results from healthcare institutions pursuing CRM patient safety programs

Alertness management and fatigue countermeasures
- State the two causes of fatigue for healthcare providers
- List the types of physical and mental errors produced by fatigue
- Discuss the effect of sleep physiology on alertness
- Discuss the effect of disrupted circadian rhythms on performance
- List the effective countermeasures to fatigue
- Discuss the proper nutrition to maintain alertness and prevent error

Team building
- Describe the benefit of teamwork to healthcare teams
- Describe the process of balancing the leader's authority with the team's participation
- List six specific actions to take to create an effective team at the beginning of the case, procedure or shift
- Assess the effectiveness of video examples of teamwork

Situational awareness: Recognizing the warning signs (red flags) of impending adverse situations
- State the history and effect of **red flag**

training in aviation.
- Define and recognize seven **red flags** unique to healthcare
- Identify **red flags** in a healthcare case study
- Provide the correct verbal response to the presence of a **red flag**

Cross-check and communication
- State the one communication technique with a proven record of decreasing communication-based errors
- Define the process of "cross-checking" performance
- State the three-step communication process for more effective team performance
- Provide an effective assertive statement to change the outcome and avoid the patient safety error in a healthcare case study

Effective team decision-making
- State the four types of decision strategies used by teams
- Utilize an effective team decision-making protocol and apply it to a healthcare problem
- List four questions to ask of the team to ensure a shared mental model
- State the most common types of decision-making errors and the strategies to avoid them

Debriefing (performance feedback)
State
- the most effective technique to transfer information to long-term memory
- three questions to ask to ensure an effective, non-threatening feedback session
- and apply the specific question to ask to ensure better performance for next time

However, the latter two industries have learned specific individual actions and teamwork skills that can mitigate the effects of fatigue on performance. High-reliability industries teach their employees how to use caffeine strategically, which foods to eat and which to avoid, and many other actions to take to fight fatigue. Remember that CRM manages the resources of the entire crew (or team) to ensure safety and mission accomplishment. Each individual's personal talents and skills are the most important resource they bring to the team; thus every individual has the responsibility to manage their "personal resources" to minimize the effect of fatigue and its impact on the team's performance and the care given to the patient. In addition, when fatigue is acknowledged, other team members can increase their vigilance and cross-check their fellow team member.

To equip the CRM project leader with a thorough understanding of the depth of the courseware, two skills will be covered in detail in this book. This discussion shows the extent of the behaviors staff and physicians should have at the completion of the initial training component of an effective CRM program.

Team building skills—what are they and how can you apply them to healthcare?

Do the following three-step activity:

1. Below, write down, either by name or title/position, as many members of your healthcare team as you can in the next 60 seconds.

_____   _____

_____   _____

_____   _____

_____   _____

_____   _____

_____   _____

_____   _____

_____   _____

(Most people in healthcare are able to write down more than 15 names/positions in one minute. [Did you remember to include the patient?] The list makes a strong point that healthcare really is a team effort.)

2. Stop for a moment and reflect on what you read in Chapter 1. In the space below write down what each of these names/positions represent to you and the team. (Hint: If humans are involved, error is inevitable.)

_____

(The answer: A potential source of error. However, if you answered this way, realize that answer is incomplete. (See explanation below.)

3. Next, in the space below, write down what these names/positions represent to you if they are properly trained in teamwork skills and use CRM safety tools.

_____

(The answer: They also represent a source of error detection and correction to trap and mitigate errors before they harm the patient.)

Effective team-building skills help ensure that your team serves as a source of error detection and correction, and not as a source of undetected, patient-harming error.

This exercise usually produces a true "aha" moment for caregivers as they realize the importance of using their team as a cross-check against errors. Their question becomes, "How can I create an effective team quickly? I may have a different team every day. I want the backup that my team provides, but I already do not have enough time in the day to do everything else I must do."

How to develop a team

The answer lies in the "best practices" of the airline industry. Although not realized by the traveling public, the pilots who fly us safely to our destinations have often never met one another prior to that flight. Nevertheless, they mesh quickly, operating together as though they have known each other for years. Surprisingly, they routinely have fewer than five minutes to conduct a team-building activity before they must attend to the task of preparing the aircraft for flight. Because no pilot knows when a catastrophic engine failure might occur or when a deadly microburst from a thunderstorm might be encountered, these team-building activities take on a critical importance. The pilots' own lives as well as the lives of their passengers depend on their expert coordination and open communication. They must "get it right," and do so quickly, or they put their flight at risk.

Many team-building activities are scripted and follow a standard protocol. Often, the flight-deck team is formed in less than two minutes' time. Our experience is that two minutes are easily found at the beginning of most routine procedures and certainly at the beginnings of most shifts, so healthcare teams may follow a similar team-building script. Organize activities with the following team-building skills:

- **Use interpersonal skills** at the most basic and common-sense level. Interpersonal skills will include the following:

  - **Introduce yourself.** It is always easier to communicate with someone you know than someone you don't know. Airlines use a flight roster with the names of the crew. Many hospitals now post the names of the staff involved in a procedure on a *white board* in the operating room (OR) to facilitate these introductions.

  - **Make eye contact.** Many studies suggest that body language conveys the bulk of the message when we communicate.[3] Failure to make eye contact when communicating robs the communicators of this important source of meaning.

  - **Support words with actions.** Actions do speak louder than words. Body language and tone will betray your real intent. A slight change in body language and tone of voice can dramatically change the message of, "Any questions?" For example, an open expression and friendly tone convey, "How can I help you with your questions?" Meanwhile, a grim, stony face and clipped tone convey, "You don't *really* have any questions, do you?"

- **Clearly provide the big picture in a "prebrief."** Flight crews always discuss the flight in general terms and then discuss specific actions at critical points expected in the flight. For example, before every takeoff, crews will brief their intended actions should an engine fail just after liftoff. The effective healthcare team leader will do the same by discussing critical decision points in the case or procedure. For example, a surgeon might announce the procedure he intends to do, highlight the critical point in that procedure, and discuss any expected contingency actions if adverse events occur at that point.

- **Invite participation from the team.** Team leaders explicitly ask team members to provide information, express their concerns, and speak up when necessary. After years of assuming that copilots would naturally speak up if they saw something amiss, and after seeing the continued disastrous effects when they didn't, commercial aviation realized that captains would have to insist, as part of their preflight team-building activities, that the comments and concerns of the copilot were important and welcomed. Today, it would be extremely rare to see a crew conduct their preflight activities and not hear a captain say to the copilot, "If you see anything that appears to be unsafe or otherwise causes you concern, please bring it to my attention immediately." Making this explicit request is necessary to break through the natural reluctance of most team members to appear to be questioning the actions of the acknowledged leader. If there is a reluctance to speak up on the part of a copilot, who often has the same level of experience and training as the captain, imagine the level of reluctance that exists on the part of nurses and other staff to express a concern to physicians. Many healthcare organizations are adding this type of safety statement to their pre-shift or pre-procedure briefings.

- **Ask questions to check understanding and begin two-way communications.** Remember that the goal of team building is to establish the free and open flow of critical information within the team. One of the simplest methods to accomplish this goal is to ask questions of the team. Questions invite a response. It's a simple pattern—I talk, you respond, and then you talk, and I respond. Thus, a pattern of response is established, and communication flows more easily.

Flight crews use this deceptively simple technique. Captains have a set of preprogrammed questions to ask of their crew to establish the information flow. For instance, a captain preparing for flight might ask his copilot, "What's the weather report?" The question invites a response. The captain must personally review the weather, but by asking that simple question about an activity related to the flight, he begins to establish the pattern of response and to open the lines of communication. With two or three more simple questions, the ice is broken, the pattern of communicating with one another is set, and the team is ready.

Physicians and other healthcare leaders can follow the example of flight crews. A few moments of thought will reveal three or four easily answerable questions that can open the lines of the communication within the team. When developing their questions, leaders should be careful to avoid asking questions that can be answered with a simple "yes" or "no." These types of questions are ineffective and do not encourage thoughtful, interactive communication. Additionally, questions should be easy, have a ready answer, and not come across as a test of knowledge or an oral examination. For example, a surgeon may ask an OR nurse, "How long has it been since you and I have done an open cholecystectotomy together?"

- **Acknowledge all communications.** Simple communication theory tells us that all effective communications are loops. When information is transferred, for the loop to be complete there must be feedback or acknowledgement (Figure 2.2). This one skill will quickly improve the effectiveness of communication. NASA research has demonstrated a clear, inverse relationship between acknowledgments and communication errors: More acknowledgements lead to fewer errors; fewer acknowledgements lead to more errors.[4] Effective leaders make it a personal habit to acknowledge every communication with either a verbal or an unambiguous nonverbal response. Like airline captains, physicians should tell their teams, "If I don't acknowledge your comment or question, assume I didn't hear it and ask it again."

With practice and forethought, a team leader can build an effective team in approximately two to three minutes by introducing herself to the members of the team, learning the team members' names, making eye contact while talking to them, providing a brief overview of the task ahead, and covering the actions to take in the most likely contingencies. The leader will ask two or three open-ended questions, acknowledge all communications, and finish up by asking explicitly for input if something looks amiss. As a result, the team will provide the leader exactly what she seeks: information to help her make the best decisions possible in the patient's care.

FIGURE 2.2

Effective communications is a loop: Questions asked by the team leader and answered by the team help establish a closed loop

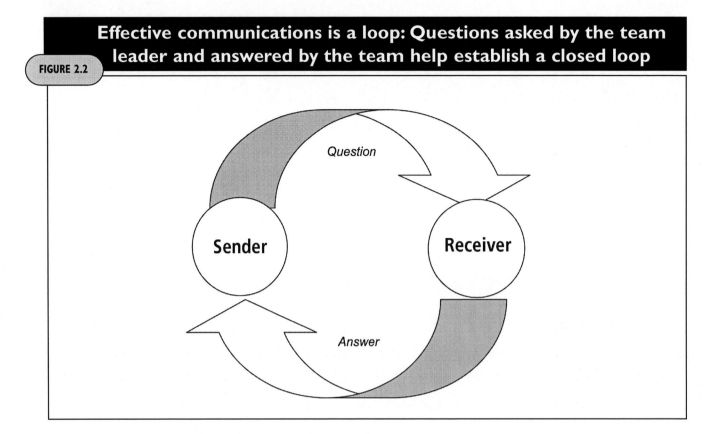

Arm your team with CRM skills

Your team won't be complete until it functions with the proper CRM skills. Encourage your team members to have an open mind when learning the new skills and to practice them for success.

Situational awareness skills—what are they and how do they apply to healthcare?

Situational awareness (SA) is a common aviation term that refers to the ability to make and maintain an accurate assessment of the "big picture" view of what is happening and to predict accurately what might happen based on what is seen at this moment. Pilots are often heard describing difficult emergency situations in terms of how much or how little SA they had at the moment. After a simulator session where a crew has had to handle both an engine on fire and a hydraulic system failure, you might hear the captain say, "So much was going on that I had low SA and didn't realize we were so close to the mountains."

Because high SA is so important for flight safety, crews spend many hours training to be able to detect warning signs that their SA is low and at risk. Being able to predict results based on current events is critical to avoiding adverse outcomes. The concept of training to recognize warning signs comes from a study of the root causes of multiple air carrier accidents. In this retrospective study, researchers analyzed scores of accidents and asked two questions:

1. Were warning signs present in the events that led up to the accident?

2. If the crew had been trained to recognize the warning signs, could they have detected them in time to avert the unwanted outcome?

Researchers realized that most aviation accidents are preceded by known and detectable warning signs. In each airline accident reviewed in the study, there were no fewer than four indicators or warning signs per accident, and in most of the accidents, seven key indicators were present. Since this landmark study, pilots and crews in both military and commercial aviation have been trained to recognize these warning signs and equipped with actions to take when a warning sign, or red flag, is detected.

Teach your team how to detect and respond to warning signs or red flags

Here is the core list of **red flags** that should be included in a training program and customized to each organization or specialty:

1. **Conflicting input:** Two or more sources of information disagree. Information may come from team members, equipment, charts, etc. For example, Air Traffic Control (ATC) alerts the flight crew that they are 15 miles from their destination airport. However, the onboard navigation equipment indicates that they are only 8 miles from the airport. If this information is not reconciled, the flight may land at the wrong airport—a decided safety risk. In a healthcare example, there have been no alarms from the pulse oximeter, but the patient's blood is very dark due to hypoxia.

2. **Preoccupation:** Fixation or intense focus on one task or problem to the exclusion of other potential dangers. Fixation or preoccupation may cause one to ignore other important priorities like flying the airplane or fighting a fire or responding to an important call. Preoccupation has contributed to

many aviation accidents, including a well-known tragedy—Eastern Airlines Flight 401—when a jumbo jet slowly descended until it crashed in the Florida everglades. The pilots were preoccupied with a faulty warning indicator. Caught up in "fiddling" with a burned out light bulb in the landing gear indicator, they were oblivious to the fact that the airplane was slowly descending toward certain death. In healthcare, fixation might lead an anesthesiologist to be preoccupied with placing an endotracheal tube while ignoring the pulse oximeter and the patient's dangerously low oxygen levels.

3. **Not communicating:** Team members do not ask for or offer input to one another. Additionally, one team member may ask another a question, but receive no reply. Note that "not communicating" does not always mean there is no talking among the team. Often, there is "talking," but no real communication. For example, comments may not be acknowledged or questions may go unanswered.

4. **Confusion:** This is a situation characterized by doubt as to what is really happening. Two behaviors are associated with this **red flag**—unanswered questions from one team member to another, and thinking, "This is stupid," "This doesn't make sense," or "Why is it/the patient doing this?"

5. **Violating regulations or standard operating procedure:** This occurs when a team member or the whole team exceeds established limits or does not follow normal procedures and no one mentions or questions the intended course of action.

6. **Failure to set/meet targets:** Examples are the easiest way to describe this red flag. Here's an aviation example: The flight plan for the flight from Memphis, TN, to Los Angeles will clearly indicate the amount of fuel required to fly that distance. At each checkpoint along the route of flight, the flight plan indicates how much fuel should be remaining in the tanks to complete the flight safely to destination. Let's say the flight plan indicates 24,000 lbs of fuel should be in the tanks as the airplane flies over Oklahoma City, but there are only 21,000 lbs of fuel in the tanks. This is a warning sign: The airplane needs 24,000 lbs of fuel to complete the flight, but only has 21,000 lbs—the target has not been met.

In healthcare, let's say that a certain surgical procedure normally requires about an hour and a half to complete. But one hour into the procedure, only one-quarter of the total, necessary steps have been accomplished. This might be a red flag. The normal time target is not being met, and that may be indicative of a more serious condition, which should alert the team to watch for other warning signs of a potential adverse outcome.

7. **Not addressing discrepancies:** This includes any unresolved confusion, doubts, concerns, and unmet targets that are not brought to the attention of the team. There is almost universal agreement in healthcare organizations that in most sentinel events and patient harming incidents, at least one member of the team was aware that something was amiss yet failed to address the issue with other members of the team.

The presence of a **red flag** does not guarantee an adverse outcome or incident. Detecting one red flag should merely alert team members to watch for the presence of additional red flags. As previously noted in the study, every aircraft accident had at least four red flags. Detecting more than one red flag in a given situation should bring the team to a heightened level of concern and awareness.

Knowing what action to take when red flags are detected is as important as recognizing them in the first place. The actions to take can be described by the statement, "See it, say it, and fix it." By "see it," we mean that team members must be trained to detect red flags and be alert for their presence. "Say it" represents the act of speaking up about what is seen and alerting others on the team to the red flag. "Fix it" means take the action needed at that moment to stop the chain of events from causing patient harm. Often, no action is needed other than to verbally note the red flag. At other times, the discrepancy causing the red flag must be fixed by specific action appropriate for the situation.

How should team skills be taught to healthcare professionals?

The answer to this question lies in the full understanding that these are "skills" or learned behaviors and actions that healthcare providers take. Aviation training designers refer to CRM as "things people do." Therefore, the skills-based seminars should incorporate these four requirements for adult learning:

- **Motivation:** Each skill module should clearly answer these questions—Why is this important to me? What is the payoff for the physician or staff member who uses this skill? How will incorporating this skill set help staff members improve their practice, provide better care for their patients, and keep their patients safer?

- **Practice:** New skills take practice. The curriculum design must allow the participants to use each of the skill they are learning or improving. This requires an instructional plan that includes case studies and other experiential activities that require participants to speak and act using the desired behaviors.

- **Reinforcement (or feedback):** CRM course facilitators must be experts at providing feedback to the participants on the use of the skills during the learning activities. Expert facilitators can discriminate among varying levels of teamwork performance and are adept at coaching participants to meet the desired skill level. Medical personnel are not typically trained to provide this level of facilitation and coaching skill. Facilitators must be chosen carefully and extensively trained. Quick train-the-trainer courses or brief periods with a consultant are not usually successful and should be viewed with caution.

- **Transfer:** What is learned in the classroom must be transferable to the hospital or clinic environment. The greatest learning transfer occurs when the fidelity of what happens in the classroom is closely aligned to the real world. In other words, the realism and accuracy of the learning activities become important to real and lasting skill improvement. Organizations choosing to work with consultants to implement CRM programs must ensure that the consultants have a depth of experience with healthcare that enables them to create learning activities with the highest fidelity to the real world of medicine.

End notes

1. N. J. Taffinder, et al., "Effect of sleep deprivation on surgeons' dexterity on laparoscopy simulator," *Lancet* 352, 1998: 1191.

2. D. Dawson and K. Reid, "Fatigue, alcohol and performance impairment." *Nature* 388, 1997: 235.

3. "Non-verbal messages in meetings," 3M. United States, Articles and Advice, *www.3m.com/meetingnetwork/readingroom/meetingguide_nonverbal.html* (accessed July 17, 2005).

4. Thomas Chidester et al., "Personality factors in flight operations: Volume 1 Leader characteristics and crew performance in a full-mission air transport simulation," NASA Technical Memorandum 102259, Moffett Field, CA, NASA-Ames Research Center, 1990.

Chapter 3

USING SAFETY TOOLS FOR PERMANENT HIGH-RELIABILITY RESULTS

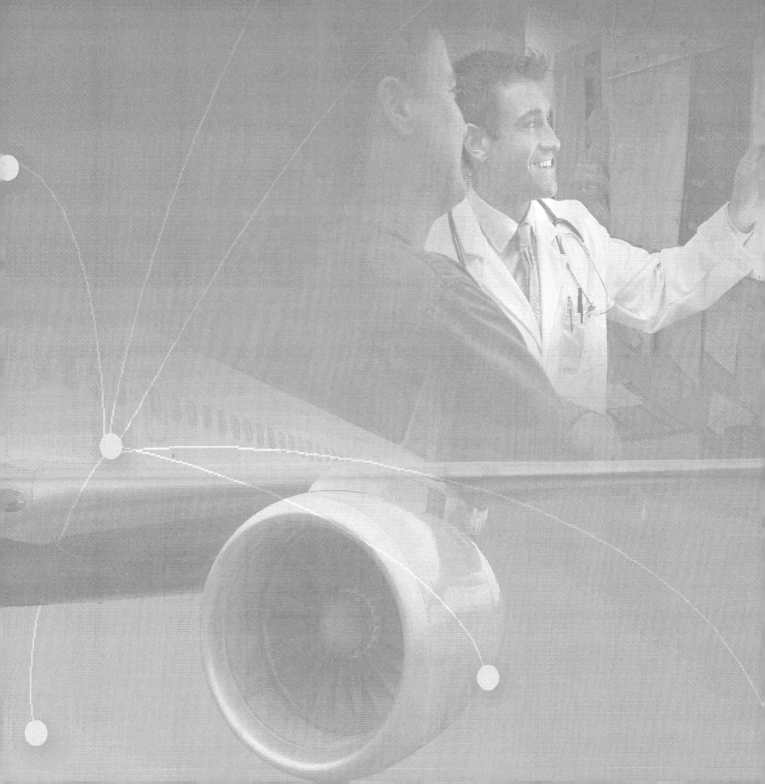

Chapter 3

USING SAFETY TOOLS FOR PERMANENT HIGH-RELIABILITY RESULTS

Why do you need safety tools in a CRM program? Why not just train the skills?

These questions will be asked by almost every healthcare organization contemplating a CRM program. The best answer to this question can be illustrated by visiting your nearest hamburger franchise and observing the operation.

System safety tools are the solution

Walk into a McDonald's anywhere in the world and order french fries. What will you get? French fries that taste exactly like the last order of McDonald's french fries—fries with remarkable consistency and taste. Fries made in New York City taste just like the fries made in Los Angeles, Tokyo, or Paris. It doesn't matter who makes the fries or where in the world they make the fries, as long as they use the "tool" that McDonald's has provided to make great-tasting fries every time.

That fries-making tool includes a checklist and the standard operating procedures to ensure that the results are consistent. Healthcare is certainly more complex than making fries, but the tools and processes necessary to achieve consistent outcomes are the same.

Tools 'hardwire' the right behaviors into the daily operating system

McDonald's, like aviation, has hardwired remarkably consistent results through its training and tools. The tools within the system control the way business is done, regardless of who does it. Outcomes are guaranteed by the system, rather than depending on staff to make "extraordinary" efforts.

Tools help make the complex become simple

The increasing complexity of healthcare makes it necessary to use safety tools. Using standardized ways of working (e.g., protocols, procedures, checklists) and communicating make it less likely that errors will occur and more likely that inevitable errors will be caught before they harm patients. Tools provide predictability for caregivers working in teams. Knowing one's specific job responsibilities and what to expect from coworkers for each situation makes it much easier to focus on one's own job while being able to back up and cross-check other team members.

Tools capture 'best practices' and ensure that all team members replicate them

Today, many healthcare processes are quite well-defined, but unfortunately sometimes they are only well-defined in the heads of a few "experts," such as a senior nurse or highly experienced physician. Recent studies show that patients receive evidence-based, consensus care about half the time. Many times, the system either falls apart or limps along at reduced efficiency when a key employee is absent because no one else really understands the game plan. Physicians may complain about not getting to practice with the "A-team." Capturing great processes and incorporating them into useful tools makes everyone an A-team member and everyone an expert. Patient outcomes and staff satisfaction improve.

Tools allow healthcare professionals to do what they do best: Apply the art and science of healing

Tools are not "cookbook medicine." Having standard plans, protocols, and tools for as many normal healthcare processes and and anticipated contingencies as possible increases the likelihood that patients will receive "best practices" care. Standardized CRM tools and processes also free up mental capacity to deal with the difficult and complex situations that require knowledge-based performance.

Tools create team ownership of performance

One of the truisms of aviation is that the copilot is just as responsible for the safety of the flight as the captain. Should the crew deviate from their assigned altitude and have a near miss or land on the wrong runway, the copilot will receive just as much enforcement attention as the captain. The safety tools used in aviation ensure shared responsibility because they require performance from all team members. Each member of the team has a vested interest in the outcome. Clearly delineated roles and processes eliminate phrases like, "Whose fault is it?"

CRM-trained healthcare professionals will eventually have a "moment of truth" when they recognize the marked difference between the old and new ways of doing their jobs. The nurse, on seeing the physician miss an important step in the procedure, perhaps due to fatigue, might previously have said nothing. But now, to prevent an adverse outcome, she speaks up with precision, just as she has been trained to do. Importantly, the physician has also been trained to hear the communication and respond appropriately. Soon, communicating in such situations becomes the norm and the patient receives the benefit. As these communications become expected and accepted, the institution's character will change and a culture of safety will be developed.

Creating a culture of safety doesn't just happen. During each moment of truth, the caregiver must choose: "Will I follow the old way or the new way"? When that moment occurs, will there be a system safety tool in place to help the nurse choose the right course of action? Will her response be hardwired? As she chooses, will she say, "This is just the way we do business here?" Effective system safety tools that help her respond this way and that hardwire the right behaviors are critical components for achieving patient safety.

Using safety tools in aviation

Checklists

Airline captains are professional pilots with years of experience. By the time a pilot is trained and certified as a captain, he or she will have made thousands of takeoffs and landings. Every one of those takeoffs and landings was preceded by a checklist. Although most airline captains could easily configure the aircraft for takeoff without the aid of a checklist, they never do so. Why? Because the consequences of a mistake can be horrendous. Missing a single checklist item, such as failing to set the flaps correctly for takeoff, can lead to an unrecoverable situation. Several fatal crashes have occurred when this step was skipped in the Preflight Checklist.

Here is an example of a preflight communication exchange between the captain and copilot illustrating the use of the checklist:

Captain: "Before Takeoff Checklist."

Copilot: "Roger, Before Takeoff Checklist." (This statement confirms that he has heard the command to run the checklist and is in fact using the correct checklist.)

Copilot: "Flaps? 15, 15, green light." (This confirms that the flap handle is correctly positioned in the 15° detent, the flap indicator gauge shows 15° on both the inboard and outboard flaps, and the cockpit light indicating that all of the flaps are correctly positioned is illuminated.)

Captain: "Checked." (Double checking that all of the above are in fact accomplished.)

Note that the pilots do not pick up a checklist, read it, and then do what it tells them. Preparing for flight, pilots quickly do what they know how to do through practice and training, and then use the checklist to verify that what they have done is correct. This is known as a "Read and Verify" checklist and takes only seconds to accomplish. This is the type of checklist that should be most often used in healthcare procedures as well. As an alternative, a checklist may follow a "challenge and response" pattern in which one team member asks a brief question and another team member verifies, acknowledges, or replies. A correctly constructed and applied checklist improves both safety and efficiency.

A third type of checklist, called "Read and Do," is used in special situations. During abnormal or emergency operations, such as an engine fire just after liftoff from the runway, pilots accomplish critical, immediate action items from memory. These are items that can't wait for the pilots to find and open the correct checklist and go to the correct page. However, once the situation is stabilized, all remaining steps will be accomplished in accordance with the checklist to ensure the absolutely correct actions are taken in this life-or-death situation. Memory items are confirmed after the fact with the checklist, and everything else is done step-by-step with the aid of the checklist. In healthcare, this type of emergency procedure could be read by a nurse, or someone not directly responding to the emergency.

No matter what type of checklist is used, all critical items on any checklist are independently verified by two cockpit crew members, and this confirmation is accomplished verbally. Pilots who fail to do this have been known to, in the stress of the moment, shut down the "good" engine and leave the engine on fire still running. Both errors quickly lead to no functioning engines.

Most healthcare facilities do not use checklists at all. Those that do often fail to use them consistently or correctly, depending too much on "Read and Do" checklists rather than "Read and Verify." Read and Do checklists are too cumbersome and time-consuming for everyday operations. All organizations implementing checklists as part of their safety tools program must understand the difference between the two concepts and design their checklists accordingly. Failure to do so wastes staff time and creates resistance from physicians objecting to "cookbook medicine."

Another common error in using checklists is the failure to crosscheck one another on the critical items on the checklist. Failure to do this greatly lessens the value of the checklist. For example, the certified registered nurse anesthetist (CRNA) reads, "Patient . . . verify ID" on the Pre-procedure Checklist and announces, "The patient is John Smith," without looking at the patient's armband. No other team members verified the announced ID with the chart or operative permit. When the inevitable wrong surgery was performed—this has actually happened—everyone asked, "What's the use of the checklist if it won't prevent the error?"

Checklists used improperly do not prevent errors

If asked, the CRNA and the rest of the team will say they accomplished the checklist. And they did say the words, but they used the tool improperly; there was no crosscheck of the information provided in response to the checklist. Checklists are an incredibly effective safety tool, but, as with any other tool or instrument, they must be designed and used correctly.

Briefings

Before every mission, flight, or simulator event, pilots and crews conduct a briefing. These short, scripted, and descriptive sessions establish a shared mental model within the team to prepare for the most likely contingencies. Most aviation organizations conduct briefings as part of a broader checklist to hardwire the briefing into normal operations. Many of the team-building skills discussed in Chapter 2 would be included in this briefing.

Debriefings

After completing a flight, pilots and crew members complete a short and highly focused discussion of key learning events from the flight. The primary goals of the debriefing are to learn from the experience, provide for continuous performance improvement, and to defuse any disagreements or tension. Effective debriefs follow a specific format: Comments should be objective and specific, focusing on what should be done differently next time to improve results or performance. Debriefings in aviation can be as short as 30 seconds, or they can last for hours depending on what is needed. Most are accomplished in two to three minutes or less.

Read Files

Airlines, like healthcare facilities, disseminate reams of information to their personnel. Some is general "nice-to-know" information; however, most is critical, need-to-know detail that affects the safe operation of airplanes. Aviation examples include Federal Aviation Administration bulletins, manufacturer's alerts, known malfunctions of en-route navigation aids, etc. Read Files consolidate this information in one place (either paper-based or Web-based) and provide a system for supervisors to know instantly if all assigned personnel have read and acknowledged (initialed) the vital information before operating the aircraft or performing the procedure.

Standard operating procedures

In aviation, every normal procedure that can be put in writing is written. Standard operating procedures (SOPs) are detailed in writing and carry the full weight of law or regulation. Training and evaluation are based on what is in the book of SOPs, and they ensure that best practices are recorded and provided to every crew member.

This is not "cookbook aviation," as pilots are given wide latitude, based on different or difficult circumstances, to deviate from SOPs as needed, as long as the departure is briefed to the team and debriefed after the event. For example, it is SOP in most airlines that pilots will make no turns just after takeoff until they have reached an altitude of at least 400 feet above the ground. However, the captain may elect to turn at a lower altitude for safety, perhaps to avoid conflicting air traffic. But he must brief his intent to turn early if he plans to or might do so, so his team is aware that this is a purposeful and safety-related deviation from SOP. After the flight, the captain must debrief his decision to depart from SOP.

Standard communication

Words have precise meanings and can affect the safety of flight operations. For instance, when setting the engine thrust for takeoff, the captain will say, "Set maximum power." The phrase "Set takeoff power" is never used. In an emergency situation and under stress, if a pilot were to use the phrase "takeoff power," it is possible the other pilot may take off or reduce power and thereby reduce thrust in a situation where more thrust is needed for safety.

Using safety tools in healthcare

Many of the safety tools used in aviation are applicable to healthcare and have been successfully adapted at multiple institutions. Some examples include the following:

Checklists

Read and Verify Checklists serve many functions in healthcare, such as these:

- Room setup
- Room turnover
- Equipment setup
- Equipment testing and maintenance
- Patient intake
- Patient checkout
- Pre-procedure charting and medical record requirements
- Testing and treatment protocols
- Blood and specimen collection procedures
- **Time-out** requirements
- Pre-procedure briefings

Tip: Virtually any repetitive process that includes items that, if missed, could have potentially harmful consequences is a good candidate for a checklist.

Briefings

These scripted team-building exercises are being used throughout healthcare facilities.

- **Pre-procedure briefings:** Conducted before any invasive procedures, these are often incorporated into a Pre-procedure Checklist and also include the JCAHO-mandated time-out items. Many institutions post team members' names on a white board in the operating room (OR) to assist in the briefing. This list includes newly hired staff, this month's fellow, or visiting medical students.

- **Shift change briefings:** Conducted at shift changes, these are accomplished by following a script devised by the staff in each department. The script (or Briefing Checklist) covers the items important and specific to that unit. Briefings identify patients on the ward or in the emergency department, succinctly specify plans for each patient, prioritize patient care, and solicit input from off-going team members about what went well and what needs attention from the incoming shift.

- **Start-of-the-day clinic briefing:** Conducted at the start of the work days, these routinely cover a review of the patients to be seen, equipment availability and function, and staffing assignments and levels for the day.

- **Intensive care unit (ICU) pre-rounding brief:** Conducted prior to rounding in the ICU, ICU briefings include a specific time and starting place, a check that key personnel are present, the order in which patients are to be seen (e.g., sickest patients, patients ready for transfer, patients awaiting diagnostic tests, patients scheduled for procedures, etc.), and specific, daily goals for each patient. A predetermined script or checklist should be used.

Most of these briefs include a "safety statement" with which team leaders explicitly invite input from the team. For example, "If anyone sees anything that is unsafe or not in the patient's best interest, please bring it to my attention immediately."

Debriefs

A debriefing, in its simplest form, should cover three points: What went well, what could be done better, and what needs to be done to address identified problems. It's important to include some acknowledgement of what went well; otherwise, debriefings will be seen as criticism and will take on a negative tone. Participation of all members of the team is important, and several approaches can be taken to minimize hierarchy. In healthcare, debriefings are not as well implemented as briefings and checklists and are frequently skipped in an effort to save time. Those institutions that have adopted debriefs have done so primarily in the OR, in ICUs at shift change, or following a code. In the OR, debriefs are often conducted as the incision is being closed. A paper or electronic form is usually completed after the debrief to capture lessons learned, record issues needing follow-up, and establish a trend database.

Debriefs should be conducted under the hospital's quality improvement/peer review program to make comments and findings "privileged" if allowed by state law. Close coordination with risk management and legal counsel is needed to ensure requirements for establishing "privilege" are met. Debriefs serve as a great learning opportunity for new hires, medical students, and house staff if handled in the spirit of continuous improvement.

An important caveat for debriefings is that items identified for follow up must be addressed. Failure to correct problems identified in the debrief will undermine the credibility of the process, and participation in debriefs will disappear quickly. It is almost better not to debrief than to raise expectations that problems will be addressed without doing so.

Read Files

Healthcare facilities use Read Files in a manner almost identical to aviation organizations. Only information critical to safe operations should be included. Often, separate Read Files are in place—one for physicians and another for staff.

Standardized communication

Many healthcare facilities are using standard communication formats. Some examples include

SBAR

The acronym stands for

- **Situation:** A brief description of the current patient situation.

- **Background:** A short recounting of the patient history and description of how the current situation came to be.

- **Assessment:** An assessment on the part of the communicator as to the severity of the situation. This assessment should follow predetermined criteria.

- **Recommendation:** A proposal for the recommended course of action.

Using this standardized communication pattern ensures the speaker is well organized in his information and gives the listener a more clear and precise picture about the current situation and the needed course of action.

Standardized patient 'hand-off' formats

Standardized communication is used to specify the exact data to be exchanged between caregivers when the patient is transferred from one to the other. See Chapter 5 for a specific example.

SOPs

The "code" scenarios used in life-support classes and Advanced Cardiac Life Support (ACLS) training are good examples of healthcare SOPs. These SOPs allow personnel to practice emergency actions, identify who will do what, and ensure that everyone understands where important equipment is located and how to use it. The protocols are written and standardized. Both training and performance are assessed, according to these written protocols on a regular basis.

Training and tools are both needed to effect lasting cultural change. Effective CRM programs provide healthcare professionals with the teamwork, communication skills, and behaviors to detect and correct errors before they harm the patient. Second, good CRM programs implement a system of safety tools that require and support the use of those error-detecting behaviors. It is the combination of training and tools that catches errors, improves efficiency, protects the patient, and provides measurable results.

Chapter 4

SETTING UP THE FOUR CRUCIAL COMPONENTS OF A CRM PROGRAM

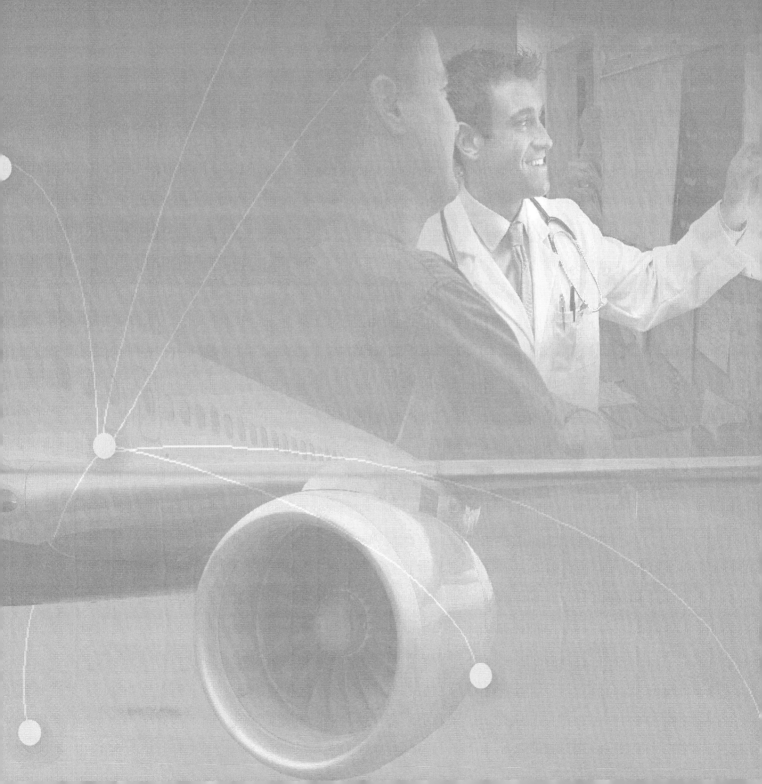

Chapter 4

SETTING UP THE FOUR CRUCIAL COMPONENTS OF A CRM PROGRAM

Four critical components of successful CRM programs

Successfully implemented CRM-based patient safety programs must follow a well-designed "flight plan." The flight plan for a successful program can be reverse-engineered by analyzing those programs in both aviation and healthcare that have produced lasting results.

First, all successful programs start with good leadership. Executives, supervisors, and managers in every successful organization are extremely busy. Therefore, to make this program work well, leaders must focus on a few, but critical, actions on top of everything else they are currently doing. These actions must be performed consistently over the course of the project. Good programs take time: Implementing a full CRM program in one large department can take up to eight months or longer, so constant leadership attention and focus are needed to avoid losing momentum or interest. The successful CRM project leader will ensure that his organization's leadership team knows what these actions are and that they are equipped to do them.

Second, the successful project leader will ensure that care providers are equipped with real teamwork and communication skills. He will design and use an effective training program to give staff the ability "to do"— to actually use specific behaviors in their daily work activities.

Third, successful CRM program leaders will ensure that those teamwork behaviors are hardwired into daily operations by creating and using processes, protocols, and checklists. These tools will become just the way business is done in the organization.

Finally, a successful program leader will prove that the project has been successful by creating and following a measurement plan. The plan will document the change in staff and physician behavior and outcomes derived from the project.

Let's take a deeper look at each of these four critical components in the flight plan for a successful CRM program:

Component #1: Good leadership

What role does leadership play? What should leaders do to ensure success?

The single most important success factor for implementing CRM is the same as any other major institutional change initiative—leadership. This cannot be overemphasized. Attempts to create the extent of change required by CRM with anything less than fully committed institutional leadership will almost certainly fail to create institutional change or produce lasting results. In this context, the definition of leadership is necessarily broad. Effort should be made to educate and enlist active support from the following four key stakeholder groups:

1. The chief executive officer (CEO), chief financial officer, chief operating officer, and key governing board members

2. Chief medical officer, chief of staff, vice president of medical affairs, chief nursing officer, chief quality officer, risk management director, etc.

3. Department heads or clinical chiefs

4. The institution's informal leaders

This latter group would include highly respected physicians, nurses, and other healthcare personnel whose opinions and advice are sought when major change is contemplated or proposed at the institution. Members of this group are often forgotten as program roll-out is planned, but their involvement is important not only for gaining agreement and commitment from the rest of the staff, but also for reinforcing support within the other leadership groups as well.

When one particular group champions CRM, it's easy to depend on that group, and to realize only later that wider support is required. For example, the CEO and chief of surgery may be excited about implementing CRM, but without comparable involvement from nursing and anesthesia, CRM implementation in surgical services will be difficult to accomplish. Likewise, involving the attending physicians and nursing staff but not the residents will create major problems. The implementation process should be reviewed frequently to be certain that involvement from the various leadership groups remains broad and reasonably well balanced.

Leadership support can be obtained and strengthened in several ways. Until CRM is more widely understood and broadly used in healthcare, it's probably easiest to introduce it to leadership by a visit to an institution that has successfully implemented CRM. An alternative is to arrange a local introductory class. This is easier to arrange, and will eventually be necessary, but it is less effective as a first step than having key leaders visit and participate directly in an ongoing CRM program. After seeing another CRM program, a next step would be holding a class or program locally with remaining leaders. Once the leadership interest has been created, a specific CRM implementation plan can be developed.

Leadership support can take many forms, so it is important to specify what is needed and to obtain commitments early in the process before moving forward. The CEO and chief of surgery may say this is a good idea, but do the individuals responsible for CRM implementation have sufficient resources, skills, and accountability? Will there be a sufficient budget to complete the initial phase of the program? Will staff be given time to undergo training and conduct tools development? Are personnel from the institution's quality improvement section available to help with measurement and tracking of implementation and desired outcomes? Will the education and training department actively assist with CRM training and implementation?

In addition to resource commitments, leaders' personal commitment to CRM must be clearly demonstrated. Will the chief of surgery participate personally in implementation? Will he or she practice CRM when operating? Will CRM become the institutional way of "doing business" or is it optional? Participation, practice, and making CRM an institutionwide standard signal that CRM is not another passing fad and will greatly improve the likelihood of successful implementation.

Requirements for time and other support should be specific. If possible, provide each leadership group with a detailed description of exactly what is required of them. For example, all participants must complete initial training of x hours. Multiple training sessions can be offered to accommodate busy schedules, but CRM training should be mandatory. If not, CRM will immediately be seen as optional. In the beginning, there is no substitute for direct, personal leadership involvement. Everyone in the classes will be looking carefully to see who is and isn't present. Having only nurses or junior physicians in the training sends the wrong message. Team members can only learn teamwork and communication skills by working with other members of the team.

Leaders must also establish, communicate, and achieve consensus on desired outcomes and success criteria for the CRM program. This requires substantive, initial leadership involvement in training and implementation. The need for establishing specific, measurable outcomes is discussed in more detail later in this chapter, but there is perhaps a more important reason for early training and involvement of leadership.

Implementing major changes in any organization inevitably creates resistance, but many of the problems and obstacles to successful CRM implementation can be predicted and proactively addressed if leadership is adequately prepared with early training and involvement in implementation. It is absolutely essential that ground rules be established early for several key issues:

Issue #1: Is this program optional or mandatory? Training classes describing results from CRM in aviation and other high-reliability organizations usually lead to easy, early acceptance of CRM concepts by most nursing and medical staff. This yields a high proportion of early adopters, and generally allows rapid initial progress. Strong commitment, highly visible involvement, and clear expectations from leadership will help win over many of the late adopters. Leadership involvement also improves direct communication with late adopters and enhances the ability to positively and consistently respond when problems occur.

Issue #2: Will you put new policies in writing? The organizational process for policy implementation can be an effective way of building consensus and informing stakeholders in the institution about the plans for CRM implementation. If the organization is unwilling to create policies to support the new CRM-related initiatives, there is great risk that the effort will fail. Changing the policies is a way for leadership to commit publicly, in writing, to the necessary changes. Here are examples of a unit-specific and generic policies:

**Consider the following sample
unit-specific and generic policies**

FIGURE 4.1

All members of the surgical services team at _____ hospital will be trained in CRM skills and are expected to use these CRM skills in their daily work and in their professional communication with other members of the healthcare organization.

All members of the _____ team at _____ will received training in CRM skills and assist in the development and implementation of CRM tools with the aim of preventing, recognizing, catching, and eliminating patient-harming errors. All team members will be expected to use these skills and tools in their daily work and in their professional communication with other members of the healthcare team.

Issue #3: Are you willing to impose consequences? In healthcare programs that require changed behavior, there are often a few physicians and staff members who do not wish to participate. Several effective approaches for getting slow adopters' cooperation are provided in Chapter 6 and Figure 6.1. These methods will help win over most of those who hold out, but you may still be left with the final 2%–3% who simply refuse to have anything to do with CRM. If one-on-one coaching, direct response to questions, and improvements to tools, etc., have not gained participation, action must be taken. Plans for this must be made in advance. CRM, after a reasonable period of development, education, solicitation of feedback, implementation, and verification of tools, etc., cannot remain optional. It must become "the way we do business," with a specific, well-publicized go-live start date.

After this date, all physicians and staff should be expected to practice their CRM skills and use the tools that have been taught and implemented in the unit. At this stage in implementation, many team members are watching to see whether leadership really is committed to implementing CRM. Failure to follow CRM policies and procedures requires specific intervention.

The nurse who doesn't use the checklists must be challenged and held accountable. The physician who insists on beginning surgery without completing the time out and briefing should not be allowed to continue scheduling and performing cases until agreeing to and performing these important pre-operative safety checks. Rapid, visible intervention should occur when a supervisor or physician responds hostilely to a staff member who expresses a patient safety concern.

It is important to have an established code of conduct that covers unacceptable behavior in a hierarchy-neutral manner. It is unlikely that anyone will speak up with a safety concern when such concerns have not been welcomed or have been met with open hostility. CRM will not lead to a culture of safety in an organization that is unwilling to support staff members who appropriately identify and communicate patient safety concerns.

Issue #4: Another issue for leadership is that of "train the trainer." To most people, this means sending someone from the education department elsewhere to learn the material and be able to give the lectures, act as a consultant, etc. Although this approach has merit, the most effective method of teaching CRM is to have the most-respected nurses and physicians practice it. These are not necessarily the oldest or most senior members of the staff, but rather the individuals whom other physicians and staff admire and would choose to care for them or their family members. Making these respected nurses and physicians experts in CRM is crucial and must be done early and deliberately. Often, they are not in official leadership positions and are not included early in implementation. They should be.

Component #2: Skills-based training workshops

Once the necessary leadership is committed, trained, equipped, and ready to guide the project to success, it's time to train physicians and staff on the specific team skills to improve coordination, communication, and decision-making. Here are several guidelines to make sure the training meets that goal:

Teach real skills. Successful CRM-based safety programs equip healthcare providers with actual teamwork and communication skills. Effective training gives your staff the ability "to do"—to actually use specific behaviors in their daily work activities. Avoid training sessions that are strictly knowledge-based. Knowledge is important to learning new skills, but not sufficient to change behavior. Courseware must be based on discrete, observable behaviors, and the training must equip staff to perform those behaviors. Make sure your leaders learn and use the skills, as well. To get the maximum buy-in from the staff, it is extremely important that your leaders support these behaviors by modeling them for the entire organization.

Train everyone who has a stake in project success. Approximately two months before the first scheduled training session make a list of the stakeholders who are the key to the success of the project. Train them first. When planning and scheduling are underway for the teamwork skills workshops, ensure that your important stakeholders, including formal leaders (executives, supervisors, managers, etc.) and informal leaders (excellent teachers, mentors, role models, and leaders without "titles"), are contacted, recruited, and encouraged to attend the first few courses.

Getting leaders trained first pays dividends. Inevitably, projects like these run into roadblocks. In the event that more funds for additional training might be needed or "naysayers" begin to resist the program initiatives, for example, getting your leaders involved early will garner their support, and they'll be more likely to give the CRM project leader the help needed to overcome these roadblocks.

Additionally, effective programs need the help of public affairs and internal communications staff to deliver the message to the rest of the organization. Include them in the first few classes. Their help in publishing project results and early successes will be invaluable to reach the "tipping point," or full acceptance, as soon as possible. Use the following outlets to spread the word:

- One-to-one communication

- General publications such as flyers, newsletter, and press releases

- Interactive exercises and public events such as seminars, educational sessions, conferences, and grand rounds

Train as teams. When conducting the teamwork skills workshops, it is best to train as a team if you work in a team. If that is not possible, either because you work in a constantly evolving team (or crew), or because you can't shut down the whole department to train as a team, ensure that you have a representative mix of physicians and staff in each session. Avoid classes that are all nurses or all physicians—especially all residents. The purpose of the skills workshops is to train team-building, communication, and coordination skills. You need complete healthcare teams to do this. The teams working together in your classroom educational activities will closely mirror the teams providing care in your organization. Each classroom team should have physician, nurse, and staff representation.

Publish the training schedule far in advance. Getting a representative mix of participants to the training sessions will require advance planning, constant attention, flexibility, and attractive benefits. Classes may need to be offered at off-peak times, including weekends. Publish the training schedule early and allow physicians plenty of time to clear their calendars and attend the sessions. Remind participants of the training schedule with e-mail and announcements during grand rounds and other departmental meetings. Additionally, sufficient time must be allowed to ensure appropriate coverage for staff and residents. Finally, never underestimate the power of offering a catered breakfast, lunch, and good snacks during the course to attract attendees.

Offer continuing education credit. Credit toward continuing medical education and continuing education unit requirements for attending the training sessions is a must. If designing your own CRM course in-house, bring your educational department into the process early to ensure that your courseware is accredited for continuing education.

Offer rewards for training. Make sure employees participating in the training are on the clock and receive pay for the time spent. Federal rules regarding payment to physicians are complex and sometimes makes reimbursement to nonemployees highly problematic. However, there are nonfinancial ways of rewarding physicians for participating in and supporting CRM efforts. For example, some malpractice insurance companies will provide discounts for CRM training. Physicians who've taken the training and practice CRM can be given priority in scheduling cases, the opportunity to work with similarly trained staff, public recognition for their efforts in improving patient safety, etc. Some type of reward system is always helpful and can usually be designed to meet a given institutions needs and resources.

Limit class sizes. Skills-based seminars with case-based, experiential learning activities work best with a minimum of 12 participants and a maximum of 48–50. Our more than 15 years' experience in providing CRM training is that a class size of 36 is optimum (See Figure 4.2). Participants should be arranged in teams around tables to facilitate interaction. The minimal team size is four participants; six to eight participants per team is more effective. Training effectiveness begins to diminish with more than 100 participants. Classes of that size make it difficult for the facilitators to provide reinforcement and feedback on the use of the skills to the participants. To accommodate classes of 48–50, close coordination with departmental leadership is needed to avoid completely shutting down the department to accomplish the training.

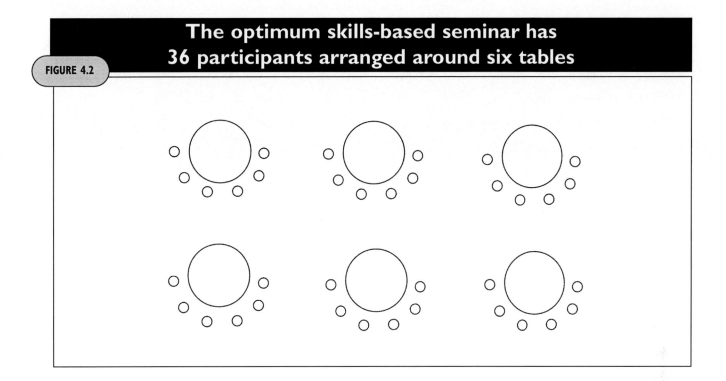

FIGURE 4.2

The optimum skills-based seminar has 36 participants arranged around six tables

Don't shorten the curriculum to save time. CRM project leaders will need to fend off requests from physicians to shorten the training. The necessary teamwork skills are deceptively simple and intuitive. Many will say, "It's just common sense!" Often, physicians will finish the training and remark, "This is great, but I could teach it in an hour." Although it may be possible to outline the content of the course in an hour, the best training sessions are case-based and require the whole healthcare team, including physicians, to maximize learning effectiveness. This can't be done in an hour. Physicians should consider the time invested in the training as a personal investment in their own skill sets and a global investment in improving the teams with which they work. In a sense, they become an extension of the class facilitator to aid the learning process for all participants.

An effective healthcare CRM course will take at least eight hours to complete. Even eight hours is dramatically shorter than similar courses in other high-reliability industries. Airline and military courses require anywhere from one and a half days to three days to complete. Many European aviation organizations require five days of training. Part of the effectiveness of the CRM courses for these organizations is based on their recognition that all the CRM skills are important. Each skill builds upon another and is a necessary part of the needed teamwork skill set.

The ideal curriculum will include at least

- fatigue countermeasures
- team-building
- effective communication
- conflict management
- situational awareness
- decision-making
- performance feedback

Each topic is taught to equip the healthcare professional with a specific and needed skill. Each skill contributes to the ability to make the best decisions in patients' care. Effective decision-making is a learned behavior and requires the complete package of skills. When well-taught, the synergy between the skills gives the provider a full skill set greater than the sum of its parts. To take advantage of this synergy, the successful CRM project leader will avoid offering a list of skills on a menu from which participants may select a la carte. Allowing participants to pick and choose according to what they feel they need will reduce the effectiveness of the program.

Ensure that participants know that training is only the first step. As important as the ideal training curriculum is to the success of the project, so is ensuring that those in training know just where the seminars fit in the overall program. Training is such a visible and tangible effort for the whole organization that many participants will see the sessions as the main event. Project leaders who have not made it clear that this educational effort is only one-half of the training and tools combination will often be asked, "How can we make this stick in our department?" All participants should know that training is just a first step in the process and should be aware that a tools-building workshop in their department will soon follow. Tools make the training stick. One way to accomplish this goal is to include in every training session an overview of the big picture for the CRM project showing the relationship of training to tools. Figure 4.3 shows an example of the type of slide that can be included in training presentations.

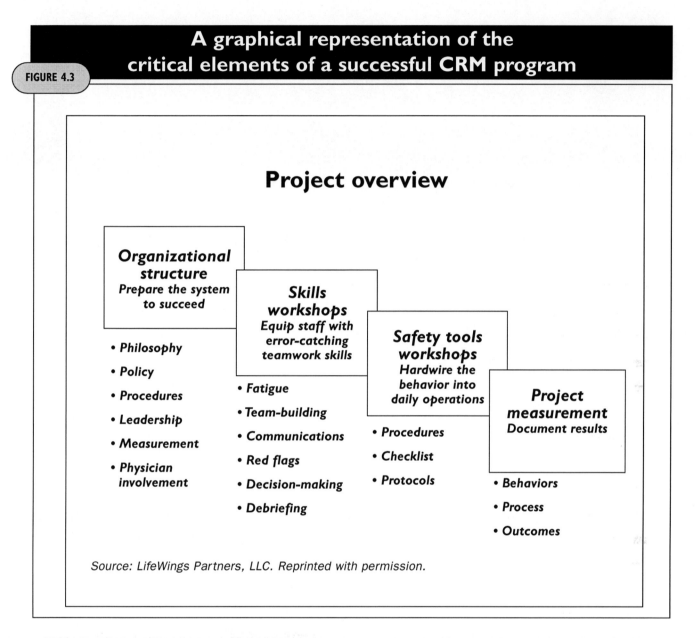

FIGURE 4.3

A graphical representation of the critical elements of a successful CRM program

Project overview

Organizational structure
Prepare the system to succeed

- Philosophy
- Policy
- Procedures
- Leadership
- Measurement
- Physician involvement

Skills workshops
Equip staff with error-catching teamwork skills

- Fatigue
- Team-building
- Communications
- Red flags
- Decision-making
- Debriefing

Safety tools workshops
Hardwire the behavior into daily operations

- Procedures
- Checklist
- Protocols

Project measurement
Document results

- Behaviors
- Process
- Outcomes

Source: LifeWings Partners, LLC. Reprinted with permission.

Train off-site. The location of the training is also important. If at all possible, get off-site. The best locations are close enough to the organization's work spaces to be convenient for the participants, but far enough from the office and patients to make it difficult to be called away in the middle of training. Training conducted on-site will suffer as participants drift off to deal with pages and calls. The success of the training depends on focus, participation, and teamwork. On-site training sessions make these difficult to attain. The temptation for participants to deal with the tyranny of the urgent is just too strong. Participants may initially resist off-site training, but once the workshop is complete, they will recognize that it was the better way to go.

CRM training programs

This section contains a lot of advice about CRM training programs. To keep it manageable, remember these simple rules:

1. Train specific skills. Ensure that the program teaches discrete, observable behaviors.
2. Train all of the skills. Don't pick and choose to save time.
3. Train all of the stakeholders, not just the care providers.
4. Train as teams.
5. Training and tools are both necessary to produce real results.

Component #3: Developing and implementing safety tools

No matter how comprehensive, applicable, integrated, and well-delivered, training alone cannot create a safe system. Providing trainees with personal skills and introducing the concepts of teamwork and using all available resources are necessary to set the stage for improvement, but this is not sufficient to change the ingrained behaviors of the larger group. All high-reliability organizations "proceduralize" safe operations using specific tools to make it easy for people to do the right thing and difficult to make an error. For instance, aviators are taught not only to communicate their intentions to Air Traffic Control, but also to use a specific way to transmit that information so it is correct, concise, and complete.

Embedding specific error-prevention or mitigation processes—or tools—in a healthcare setting ensures that problems not only get fixed today, but also that they stay fixed. Additionally, the exercise of developing tools using the standardized methods borrowed from more-experienced high-reliability organizations teaches the team to create solutions that are consistent across the institution. It is imperative that tools be customized to address the safety concerns and workplace operations of a specific unit—just as each airplane type must have a specific checklist for its unique equipment and mission. However, if a standard format is used across the hospital, a nurse will recognize the form and function of a similar tool used in another unit. The benefit of creating and following a flexible template across an institution (and perhaps eventually across the spectrum of healthcare arenas) allows personnel to gain technical competence quickly when moving across departments. Understanding the basic concept of creating tools gives the entire team a better idea of what the tools are meant to accomplish and gives them the knowledge to continue tool creation independently of a trainer or consultant. A familiar system with good ideas incorporated from other departments will improve efficiency, make the training of new hires easier, and hardwire error-catching behavior into the daily operations of the unit. It will become "the way we do business."

In this section, we will present a basic road map for developing tools. A hypothetical hospital unit, a composite based on the experience of the authors in working with various departments across many institutions will be used as an example to illustrate the steps in the process. This is how work might progress in a busy catheterization lab:

Step #1: Uncover hidden areas of risk

To design the most useful tools, first identify the most pressing issues for the healthcare unit. An excellent method for doing this is to perform a Safety Climate Survey. There are several previously piloted and validated surveys available from national safety organizations (e.g., the Agency for Healthcare Research and Quality at *www. ahrq.org* or from *Culture at Work in Aviation and Medicine by Helmreich and Merritt,* 1998, pp. 257–260), or a unit may want to develop its own tools.

In addition to asking about specific unit concerns, Safety Climate Surveys can uncover more general problems such as poor coordination between units, lack of management support for safety, punitive error-reporting systems, etc. A few open-ended questions may encourage team members to recommend solutions to problems. Areas of strength may also be uncovered upon which the project can capitalize.

Cath lab example:

Physicians and staff survey results indicate there is strong support for safety from institutional and departmental leaders. But there is poor communication within the team, particularly with authority figures, and a tendency to cut corners when things are busy.

Step #2: Identify and prioritize specific needs with unit personnel

Next, convene a brainstorming session of a representative cross-section of people from the unit, including physicians, nurses, and other staff members. Choose subject matter experts—those with extensive daily operational experience, a history of insight, and motivation for improvement. The selected team should first review the results of the safety survey. Then, in a forum where all input is respected, thoughtful questions can uncover specific departmental areas of concern. In addition to readily identifiable unsafe processes, the team should identify process "workarounds." Clever, creative, and well-motivated people frequently develop workarounds to get the job done despite system deficiencies, but these quick fixes often create risk. Only by providing the opportunity to identify these faulty processes will these specific issues be brought to light. Once items are identified, they must be prioritized and vetted by leaders.

Cath lab example:

In their work group meeting, personnel identified these specific needs (in order of priority):

1. Improvement in communication between physician and staff

2. Improvement in coordination during procedures (e.g., "I do my job well but don't really coordinate with others well, and don't really understand what others are going to do")

3. Discrepancies between scheduled and performed procedures (e.g., "The physicians frequently don't tell us whether the planned procedure has changed and we don't have the equipment for the new procedure")

Step #3: Match available tools to specific needs

Once the team members have identified and prioritized the issues, they begin the process of hardwiring safety processes into daily operations. Properly designed, these safety tools will make it easy to do things right and difficult to do things wrong via a standardized system of processes and procedures that eliminate dependence on personal memory, initiative, or workarounds.

At this point the team must learn about the tools that aviation and other high-reliability organizations have used to address problem areas. Attending a short course by someone with experience developing and using these kinds of tools is invaluable (see *www.SaferPatients.com*). A good understanding of the highly polished content and formatting used by these organizations will allow the tools team to have a clear view of what it is trying to accomplish.

Cath lab example:

The cath lab team attended a presentation by CRM consultants with experience designing checklists and processes. The team matched the most appropriate tool to their high-priority safety issues. They chose a pre-procedural briefing.

Step #4: Seek leadership approval for the work

At this point the team must do a "reality check" with unit or departmental leadership. Leaders with a larger view of their area and an understanding of the concerns of the entire institution may reprioritize or broaden the scope of the work. It is also important to ensure that leadership supports the work of the team and agrees that all personnel will use the tools, once developed and refined. No stronger message can be sent than when a knowledgeable leader commits to becoming an expert on the tool, agrees to model the change in behavior once the work is completed, and sets the policy for departmental use of the tool.

Step #5: Create tool content

Initially, the content of the tool must be mapped out. The team writes down all the things that are to be accomplished with or included in the tool. At this point, order and wording are not important, only that all the necessary requirements are captured.

Cath lab example:

The cath lab wants to

- know the names of all the team members in the procedure room—a first step to working as a team

- verify patient identification and planned procedure and include a discussion of potential problems

- have an understanding that everyone is expected to speak up if they need clarification or see anything unsafe

- ensure that all personnel and equipment are ready before starting the case

As they work on the checklist, the team also identifies the need to emphasize when additional precautions should be taken for bloodborne illnesses and that the operative permit is correct and signed. Although these items were not discussed in Step #3, the process of creating the tool uncovered the need for them.

The checklist addresses each of their four issues. It requires the cardiologist to invite team members to speak up and requires him to state the planned procedure. Team members must verbally verify that equipment is available. Finally, all team members are required to participate in the briefing, and this allows them to coordinate their activities.

Step #6: Format the tool

The checklist will exist in two forms: the expanded checklist and the checklist. First, create the expanded checklist. This form of the checklist provides detailed information on who, what, when, and why. This is an excellent tool for teaching new hires and staff why certain steps are included and what they mean. This form of the checklist is not used in daily operations, but rather for training and reference only.

Next, the verbiage must be whittled down to the briefest and most concise terms to create the checklist used on a daily basis. The "challenge and response" type of checklist (Chapter 2) works well to verify completion of a multi-step process and was chosen by the cath lab team for part of their pre procedure time out.

Cath lab example:

One step in the expanded format of the cath lab checklist was, "Physician announces complete procedure he or she plans to do, and nurse confirms that this is the procedure agreed to on the Op Permit." The final version of the step reads, "Procedure . . . State (MD); . . . Confirm from Consent (RN)." An example of an expanded checklist and the final format are shown in figures 4.4 and 4.5.

Step #7: Test the tool

Next, have someone not on the original development team try the tool. Are the steps concise, understandable, and in the right order? How much and what kind of training is required to use the tool? Are there other components that should be included? Sometimes difficulties are uncovered that were not apparent when the team was sitting around a conference table. The tool can be updated when the test is complete.

Cath lab example:

Staff discovered a hand-held checklist would not work as the person designated to use it was gloved. A wall-mounted checklist was subsequently designed and installed.

Step #8: Demonstrate the tool

The refined tool is now ready for demonstration to the rest of the unit leadership and staff. Everyone must understand the issues originally identified and how the tool addresses one or more of the high-priority issues. Inputs from the larger organization can then be incorporated.

Cath lab example:

No changes were needed and the checklist was approved for use.

Cath Lab Preprocedure Briefing Expanded Checklist

FIGURE 4.4

Names of Team on White Board_____**Checked (RN)**
Nurse should write names of all team members on the white board and introduce any new members at the start of the case.

Patient Name . . . . **State (MD)**
. . . . **Confirm (RN)**
Physician should state the patient's name and the nurse, who confirmed patient's identification from chart, armband and patient, confirms name (at least two separate sources of identification).

Procedure . . . . **State (MD)**
. . . . **Confirm from Consent (RN)**
Physician announces complete procedure he/she plans to do and nurse confirms that this was procedure agreed to on the Op Permit (two sources of verification).

Adverse Patient Hx/Allergies . . . . **Request (MD)**
. . . . **Respond from Chart (RN)**
Physician requests nurse to review from patient's chart any pertinent adverse history or allergies.

Single or Double Glove? . . . . **Request (MD)**
. . . . **Respond (RN)**
Physician requests from the nurse whether there is the need to double glove and be cautious because the patient has a blood-borne disease.

Equipment . . . . **Available and Checked (RN)**
. . . . **Available and Checked (Scrub)**
Both the nurse and scrub tech verify that equipment they are responsible for is in the room and has been checked for operability.

Invitation to Speak Up . . . . **from script (MD)**

"If any member of the team sees anything that is unsafe, I expect you to speak up."

In order to standardize and explicitly state this responsibility, a succinct script has been developed and will be stated before the procedure starts.

"Is the Team Ready?" . . . . **Respond ("Nurse", "Scrub" etc.)**
If each member of the team is ready, he/she quickly states his/her position. If not prepared to proceed, state, "Stand by" and advise when ready.

"Briefing Complete" . . . . **Complete (MD)**
Physician states briefing complete and ready to start case.

Cath Lab Preprocedure Briefing

FIGURE 4.5

Names of Team on White Board_____ Checked (RN)

Patient Name_____ State (MD)
_____ Confirm (RN)

Procedure_____ State (MD)
_____ Confirm from Consent (RN)

Adverse Patient Hx/Allergies_____ Request (MD)
_____ Respond from Chart

Single or Double Glove_____ Request (MD)
_____ Respond (RN)

Equipment _____ Available and Checked (RN)
_____ Available and Checked (Scrub)

Invitation to Speak_____ (from script – MD)

"If any member of the team sees anything that is unsafe, I expect you to speak up."

Is Everyone Ready?_____ Respond ("nurse", "scrub" etc.)

Briefing_____ Complete (MD)

Step #9: Establish a written policy for checklist use and set a start date

Unit leadership should decide when the tool is ready for general use, publish a letter of instruction that mandates the use of the tool, and subsequently revise the policy and procedures manual. Leadership should also designate a checklist owner with the responsibility for capturing and incorporating subsequent revisions according to a preestablished process and schedule. Failure to designate an owner and revision process will cause needed changes to be lost, use of the checklist will decline, and ultimately workarounds will appear that undermine the intended purpose of the tool.

Cath lab example:

Nurse Jeff Cohen is designated as the checklist owner. Issues raised during cath lab debriefings relative to the checklist are recorded and given to Jeff to analyze trends and comments. The original cath lab tools team was formally assigned to meet every six months and incorporate approved revisions into the checklist.

Component #4: Measurement and documentation of results

With trained leadership, effective skills training, and hardwired safety tools in place, how do you make sure the project produces results? Follow the measurement plan created at the beginning of the project. Use these guidelines to design an effective measurement plan for CRM projects:

Obtain leadership support for measurement

Measuring to document the results of the CRM program is a significant undertaking for any organization. Data collection requires the effort of both support staff and caregivers. Effort expended on measurement often is seen as an additional activity, tangential to the primary task of taking care of patients, and therefore approached with a lack of enthusiasm. Many organizations do not collect the baseline data they need to prove the results of their project and will discover they need additional data collection, over and above what is presently done. This extra effort and any additional data-collection burdens require the strong support of leadership and their constant attention to make sure measurement gets done.

Define success for this project. When designing the measurement plan for the CRM project, one of the most important steps is to identify the factors that define success. Once identified, CRM project leaders must gain agreement from the stakeholders on the success criteria. This part of the measurement plan must be accomplished before training starts, especially if the measurement plan calls for a pre- and post-project comparisons.

Conduct measurement plan interviews. An effective method to reach agreement among stakeholders is to conduct a series of 15–20 minute one-on-one interviews with them. In these interviews, ask these three questions:

1. *How much do you know about the CRM project?*

   This is an important question. Those interviewees who don't know about the project will need to hear a brief description of it. Include in this overview the program's purpose, components, and scope. For those who do know about the program, ask them to describe it in their own words and then fill in any gaps in their knowledge.

2. *At the end of the project, what has to have happened for you to consider the project a success?*

   Essentially, you are asking the interviewee to visualize the end state in their department. What does the department look like when the project is complete? What do they see? Their answer will reveal what is important to them and what they want to see changed about how care is given in their organization. Expect to hear answers like, "I don't ever want to see another wrong surgery." or, "I don't want to have to deal with another sentinel event with communications as a root cause."

   Occasionally, the interviewer will have to manage expectations during these interviews. CRM programs do not cure cancer, meaning that sometimes stakeholders have unrealistic expectations about what a CRM program will do for the organization. Allowing the bar to be set too high during these interviews will only set the stage for disappointment in the results when the project is complete.

3. *For you, what would be an acceptable measure to prove that (the answer from question #2) has actually happened?*

   The first part, "for you," is a vital component of the question. For instance, let's say the interviewee answered question #2 with, "I don't ever want to see another wrong surgery." For her, the only acceptable measure might be the complete absence, for the rest of her life, of any wrong surgeries in her hospital. Anything less means, to her, the program was not successful. For another stakeholder providing the same answer, an increase in the number of days between wrong surgeries or a decrease in the number of wrong surgeries per 10,000 cases may be an acceptable measure. Remember, the aim is to seek agreement among the stakeholders on both the goals and the measures that prove the goals have been met.

Often stakeholders can be confused about the difference between an "outcome measure" and a "process measure." An outcome measure is something like "fewer wrong surgeries." A process measure is something like an "increase in compliance with the time-out briefing requirement." If the respondent provides a process measure as their answer to question #3, the interviewer should point out the difference and ensure that the respondent will be satisfied in the end with that particular measure as proof of the project result. Clarifying the difference may help avoid arriving at the end of the project only to have that stakeholder say, "The fact that we have greater compliance with our time-out briefing [the measure] doesn't really prove we have fewer wrong surgeries [the goal]."

Once you have conducted all of the interviews, collate your answers and display them in a way that allows synthesis of the results. Then decide where there is agreement on the expected results. Consider these pointers about this process:

1. Ask, "Who is the most important stakeholder or stakeholders? Who will cast the most votes as to whether the project was a success?" Once identified, weigh their answers accordingly.

2. Look for goals that you know the program can accomplish. Determine these by being familiar with other CRM programs and the results they have achieved. Emphasize those in the final measurement plan. This is not to say don't have "stretch goals," or other high expectations, but be realistic in what can be accomplished and create the expectation for success.

3. The organization will typically want to publish its successes in periodicals and peer-reviewed journals. As the measurement plan is finalized, keep an eye toward this goal and ensure that data that support this aim will be collected and analyzed.

4. Scrub your results and compare them against the following four levels of measurement by Kilpatrick:

   Level I—Reaction evaluation. Did the participants find the training useful and relevant to their jobs? Did they change their attitudes as a result of training?

   Level II—Learning evaluation. Did the participants learn anything? For example, as a result of the training, can the learner accurately make an assertive statement?

   Level III—Behavior evaluation. Are the skills actually being used in the workplace? For example, can we document evidence that physicians and staff are communicating more frequently or more effectively?

Level IV—Results evaluation. Does the organization reap the harvest of the investment in the program in terms of improved outcomes, such as fewer wrong surgeries?

Levels III and IV are the most important types of evaluation for performance-based training. Level III evaluations assess on-the-job application of acquired knowledge and skills. Level IV assesses whether organizational outcomes are enhanced as a result of the knowledge and skills acquired and applied.

Does the measurement plan provide for all four levels? If not, determine what data must be collected to measure each level. Clearly, levels III and IV will be of the most interest to the stakeholders and deserve the bulk of the measurement effort.

Figure 4.6 may help you organize your measurement plan and ensure that a thorough picture of the project results is created.

One of the major byproducts of using this process to create the measurement plan is that unity of purpose among organizational leadership grows and stakeholders begin to take ownership of the project. Something remarkable happens when stakeholders are asked their opinion about goals, results, and measures. The simple act of asking, "What do you think?" creates enthusiasm, buy-in, and support among those who will most influence the outcome of the project. It is a powerful tool for project success.

An overview of the four levels of measurement

FIGURE 4.6

Sample Assessment and Evaluation Strategies

Level	What is analyzed?	What we want to know	Assessment Method	*What the Client Will Learn*
1. Reaction	• Course design • Cultural climate of the hospital toward Patient Safety	• Usefulness • Relevancy • Does a culture of Patient Safety exist?	• Critiques (CQ) • Safety Climate Survey (SCS)	• (CQ) Did the learner find the training useful and interesting? • (SCS) Did the cultural and operational climate toward patient safety improve as a result of the training?
2. Training	Is subject matter effectively delivered to learners?	• Are attitudes shaped?	Human Factor Attitude Survey	• Did the training cause an attitude shift in the learner toward the use of team skills? • Attitude shift is indicative of performance change.
3. Behavior	Did learners translate training into workplace performance?	• Are new skills/behaviors being used in the workplace?	• Performance Assessment Form (PAF) • Critical Incident Reports (CIR) • Focus Group Interviews (FGI) • Annual Performance Reviews (APR)	• (PAF) Do trained observers see the application of the skills in the workplace? • (CIR) Are the skills being applied and did the application prevent errors? • (FGI) Are the skills being applied and did the application prevent errors? • (APR) Do staff demonstrate the use of the new skills?
4. Results	Did the hospital reap the harvest of improved workplace performance?	• Have quality care and patient safety improved? • Are there fewer errors and sentinel events? • Are there fewer open claims? • Has efficiency improved?	• Patient Satisfaction Surveys (PSS) • Wrong surgery avoidance • Medication error reduction • Error Reporting (ER) (reduction in all types of reportable errors/near misses)	• (PSS) Did Press-Ganey scores improve as a result of the training? • (ER) Were specific errors reduced as a result of the training?

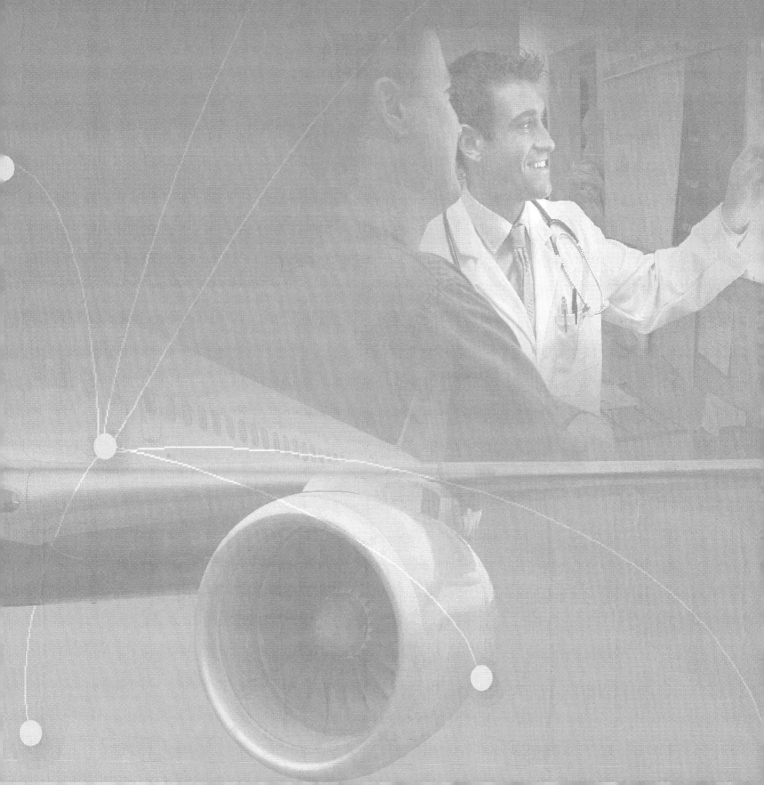

Chapter 5

HARDWIRING FOR SUCCESS:
EXAMPLES OF USEFUL SAFETY TOOLS

5

HARDWIRING FOR SUCCESS: EXAMPLES OF USEFUL SAFETY TOOLS

In this chapter, specific examples of safety tools for healthcare will be illustrated and discussed. Creating a well-written checklist or briefing guide is not as simple as it might appear. Poorly designed tools create resistance from users and prevent implementation. Users will not see any improvement and may actually experience decreased efficiency with poorly constructed tools. This may lead to the conclusion that CRM doesn't help. For these reasons, it is important to know the difference between effective and ineffective tools.

Effective vs. ineffective tools

A well-constructed checklist is much more than simply a laminated version of the printed procedure. The Joint Commission on Accreditation of Healthcare Organizations (JCAHO)–mandated **time-out** checklist (Figure 5.1) is difficult to read. It is all capital letters and contains considerable verbiage strung together, making it impossible to keep one's place on the list. To perform the briefing crisply, the listed components would have to be memorized, and this would lead to nonstandard performance, difficult training, and missed steps (as often occurs with over-reliance on memory).

Also, the topics are vague, which leads to variability and questions. Should the physician cover all the patient's medical problems or only the pertinent ones? What should the anesthesiologists say when they get to the term, "etc."? Without clear and definitive answers to these questions, each briefer would perform this checklist differently, sometimes leading to a rambling monologue of unneeded information. Note that the instructions state that the proceduralist "announces" the patient information. If any of that information is

An example of an *ineffective* safety tool for a JCAHO Time-Out Briefing

FIGURE 5.1

"TIME-OUT" BRIEFING CHECKLIST

DO NOT USE

CHECK

PHYSICIAN ....ANNOUNCES THE PATIENT'S
     NAME, DIAGNOSIS, SURGICAL PROCEDURE, SITE AND
     SIDE, NEEDED IMPLANTS AND STUDIES, POSSIBLE
     COMPLICATIONS, MEDICAL PROBLEMS

ANESTHESIOLOGIST.............GIVE STATUS ON HOW
     SEDATION OR INDUCTION WENT, AVAILABILTY OF
     MEDICATIONS, BLOOD, ETC.

NURSE.................................ADVISE THAT THE CASE
     CAN START AND REMIND EVERYONE TO BE SAFE,
     MEDICATIONS, BLOOD, ETC.

wrong, it may not be caught. Information provided by this checklist is not formally verified by any other source, (i.e., there's no crosscheck). The checklist implies the nurse will give the go ahead to start the case after the time out is over, but is the rest of the team ready? Telling everyone to "be safe" is like saying, "Try harder." Healthcare workers are already working very hard and doing their best to be safe. They need tools and systems to help them be safer, not admonitions.

Last, there are check boxes to indicate that the steps were completed. Why is this necessary, and how are the data collected from these boxes? If a paper-based system is used, a fresh checklist will be needed for every case. Unless there is a good reason for obtaining this information, requiring a written check-off of the steps is unnecessary.

The cath lab pre-procedural briefing checklist (Figure 4.4) from the last chapter is an example of a concise and useful tool. This checklist is brief and to the point. Each step is a cue to a specific action and designates to whom the step belongs. In a large font, a laminated version of this guide can be put on the wall for the cardiologist to read as he or she gowns and gloves. It is intuitive. Once it is demonstrated to the team, it can be easily performed with little additional training. There is no need to memorize anything, yet all important steps are completed. All members of the unit use the same format, so anyone who is assigned to a particular room is prepared and knows what to expect. The entire checklist can be accomplished in less than two minutes.

It concisely addresses all of the concerns identified by the team during the tools development process. Team members will know each other's names, which is especially important for teaching institutions where house staff and fellows rotate frequently. Addressing someone by name improves interpersonal relations and the communication necessary to build a good team. It is also a better way to get someone's attention if problems occur, rather than making an undirected, general statement. The briefing itself opens the dialogue between physicians and staff.

The JCAHO's time out requires that the patient's name and procedure be verified. This briefing reminds the team to use two sources of information for verification. The physician states the patient's name. The nurse confirms that patient's identification by checking the chart and the armband and by asking the patient. Then, the physician specifies what procedure she plans to do, and the nurse verifies that with the consent form. This is a good example of crosschecking.

There is a tendency to hear what one expects to hear and not to question the statements of an authority figure. If the physician's custom is to announce the patient's name and procedure without crosscheck, there will be a strong tendency for everyone to agree from ignorance or deference, and this can be a source of misidentification. Remember the nurse in the near-miss event described in Chapter 1? She asked the patient "Is your name Reynaldo?" rather than asking him to state his name. She negated the built-in crosscheck process. Building cross-check and redundancy into the verification process eliminates the errors that occur from depending on a single source for correct information—but the cross-check process must be used.

In preparation for the cath lab procedure, the nurse reviews the chart and has access to it as the physician begins the prebrief. The physician asks the nurse to summarize patient history that may cause problems and then fills in any additional information that might be useful for the team. This prepares the team for contingencies. Finally, the team leader stresses that it's everyone's responsibility to speak up if they see anything unsafe. An explicit statement is far more effective in setting expectations for all team members than assuming that everyone will understand this responsibility.

There is a final check that all needed equipment is available and operational and that everyone is ready to start the case. This final question reinforces the concept of team by showing respect for the team members and acknowledging that their activities are important to providing the safest and best care for the patient. In addition to improved patient safety, careful preparation of an effective, correctly designed checklist standardizes the procedure. Standardization leads to increased efficiency by eliminating error, delays, and rework.

In summary, both the content and the format must be correct to make the tool maximally useful and effective. A tool that is not helpful and concise will rarely be used. Poorly designed tools create the danger that the entire concept of using CRM and safety tools will be discarded as "not applicable to healthcare."

When one understands the design and logic behind simple tools such as checklists, briefings, debriefings, and data transfer formats, it isn't difficult to build a basic tool set. But ignore format, design, and style guidelines at your peril. Poor tools put your program at risk. Here are some examples of a few, specific, well-designed safety tools:

White board

Background: Military flying squadrons frequently use dry-erase white boards throughout their operational spaces. Flight schedules, aircraft assignments, crew member rosters, emergency procedures, and weather reports are just a few of the items that are routinely posted on white boards throughout the squadron. The intent is to share as much information as possible with as many people as possible. The goal is to develop a shared mental model between team members of what's happening, what will happen, and the operational environment for the flight.

A simple dry-erase white board mounted on the wall in a procedure or operating room (OR) can accomplish the same goal in healthcare. Loaded with pertinent information about the team or procedure, white boards serve as an excellent quick-reference source.

Methodology: Determine what information is needed at a glance by asking the unit's team members and create permanent headers or titles for those data on the unit's white board. Rub on letters, available from a hobby shop, work well to create these headers. In terms of data, just enough to do the job is best. Although considerable information can be packed onto a large board, it is best to keep the information to a useful minimum. Remember, the board must be redone for every case and a plethora of data makes locating any one piece of information difficult. Figure 5.2 below shows an example of a simple format for general surgery:

An example of a white board, mounted on the wall in the OR

WHITE BOARD
Used to improve coordination and communication in an OR

TEAM

Surgeon

1st assistant

Scrub tech

Circulator

Anesthesiologist/CRNA

Others (name/position)

PATIENT INFORMATION

Name

Procedure

Site/side

Studies

Implants

Allergies

Blood type

The board lists the names of the people in the room. Physicians often express gratitude for this simple feature, as they often forget names of people with whom they work infrequently and are sometimes embarrassed to ask. This may be the only way housestaff can know the nurses and techs by name and vice versa. If there is a new person observing the case, communication is better when all know that person's name and reason for being there.

Basic data about the patient are also written on the board. However, remember that the patient's record is the definitive source for most information. Using the transcribed information on the white board as the single source of information to make critical decisions is discouraged because incorrect transcription can be a source of error.

Use the white board data to cross-check all the information required for the formal time out: patient's name, procedure, site, side, studies, and implants. Use the studies and implant data as a memory aid to ensure these are in the room. This is important for cases that require these, and will avoid delays. The white board data are also a quick reference about allergies and blood type so that if medications or blood products are ordered, any team member can cross-check the accuracy of the order. Anyone entering the room can check the board for basic information.

Customize the white board for specialized procedures. For instance, an orthopedic surgeon may want to list the time the tourniquet was inflated. A cardiac surgeon might want to know the time the patient went on bypass. In pediatric surgery, the weight of the patient might be an important thing to include. These items can have permanent headers on the board for department wide requirements or can be written on the board with a dry-erase marker for individual physician preference.

For hospitals with electronic medical records, it is possible to create an electronic white board. Information from the patient's chart can be imported to the board, eliminating transcription error and shortening room turnaround time.

Debriefing guide

Background: Aviators conduct a performance feedback session after a flight mission. This is a core CRM practice for them. During this session, all team members involved in the flight will discuss what happened and what can be learned to improve performance for next time. A carefully constructed script, or guide, is followed (see Figure 5.3). This script keeps the discussion on point and precisely targeted to the most essential action steps needed to improve outcomes.

These sessions normalize the discussion about effective and ineffective performance. The habit of performance feedback allows critique without emotional content. It's just the way business is done to get better. Also, these sessions provide a mechanism to close the loop on conflict among team members and keep the lines of communication open for next time.

FIGURE 5.3

An example of a Debriefing Checklist

Debriefing Checklist

1. What went well?

2. What should we do differently to improve for next time?

3. Did we have everything we needed to do our job?

Debrief Checklist complete.

Submit paper debriefing record.

Source: LifeWings Partners, LLC. Reprinted with permission.

These sessions are commonly called "debriefs" by pilots. Debriefs in high-reliability organizations can take as little as 30 seconds and as long as one hour. For most commercial aviation and healthcare applications, debriefs normally take from 30 seconds to three minutes. The length is determined by the complexity of the event, the time available, and the lessons that need to be learned.

Methodology: Most healthcare organizations conduct debriefs in the intensive care unit (ICU) or at the end of a shift in the emergency department (ED). However, the concept can be applied anywhere in a healthcare organization. Our discussion of this example will be centered upon the OR. When conducted in the OR, the debriefing format, or script, is often posted on the wall for ready reference. Additionally, a paper-based form corresponding to the wall-mounted guide will also be used to capture, in writing, significant items of discussion.

To use the debriefing guide effectively, the healthcare team accomplishes the following steps:

1. At the appropriate time, usually as the incision is being closed, the team lead will call for the "debriefing checklist." Normally, the team leader is the surgeon, but for purposes of the debrief, the circulator or other team member can call for and conduct the checklist. It is important for all members of the team to be present and participate.

2. One member of the team will be designated to act as the unit "scribe" to capture significant discussion on the paper-based debriefing form.

3. The team leader will refer to the wall-mounted checklist and ask the first question on the script, **"What went well?"** Team members may answer only by exception; there is no need to say anything if they have nothing of significance to add. Or some institutions require all team members to provide an answer. We recommend that all team members be required to participate. To encourage participation, the most junior team member goes first, and then each team member answers in turn. The team leader responds last.

4. The team leader will then ask the next question on the checklist, **"What should we do differently to improve for next time?"** The focus should be on personal performance issues, including teamwork, communication, coordination, and technical skill. Again, team members might answer only by exception or in sequence by team seniority, most junior to most senior. Significant performance improvement items should be annotated on the paper-based form.

5. When discussion is complete, the team lead will move on to the next item on the checklist, **"Did we have everything we needed to do our job?"** This question deals primarily with equipment issues and is used to tweak the system to ensure needed equipment is always in place, tested properly, and operable. Again, it is vitally important that any significant discussion in response to this question is recorded on the paper-based form for follow-up. If identified issues are not corrected, personnel will soon stop debriefing.

6. The team lead will announce, **"Debrief Checklist complete,"** when discussion is finished.

7. The paper form is dropped off at a central collection point to be gathered at the end of the day for analysis. This step is included on the checklist to ensure that it is not forgotten. Discussion items recorded on the form will be entered into a database for trend analysis and to provide a mechanism for follow-up on items needing attention.

Using this system has several byproducts. Essential communication and coordination skills are hardwired into daily operations. Additionally, when properly conducted, conflict is resolved and barriers to communication among the team members are removed. Most important for the team, a well-designed debriefing system with adequate and consistent follow-up will prevent the same problems from happening repeatedly. This creates a tight cycle of improvement leading to a consistently better quality of care.

IMSTABLE, a standardized data transfer format

Background: Flawless transfer of information between combat pilots and troops on the ground is absolutely critical. Errors in their communications can lead to deadly "friendly fire" accidents. Few things are more tragic than the needless loss of life when fliers drop ordnance on their own soldiers, mistaking them for the enemy due to poor communication. Military aviators use a specific communication safety tool to avoid these errors when communicating with ground troops. It's called a Nine Line Transmission.

Ground troops vector the pilots onto enemy positions with a radio transmission that contains nine specific parts, or lines. Each line contains exacting detail and is always given in the same order and sequence. Every communication, in practice and real combat, is given in this sequence. The sequence is practiced thousands of times between soldiers and pilots. If any information is missing, or doesn't make sense, the pilot will instantly know it. Then the pilot can seek clarification or abort the bombing run to avoid tragedy.

Transfer of patient data among caregivers is also an error-prone process. Often, nurses give quick verbal reports, especially when time is of the essence. Figure 5.4 is an example of a form designed with the same principles used in a Nine Line Transmission. It keeps patients safer by ensuring that all the data about critically ill patients are captured and transmitted to other members of the team.

Methodology: Staff use this form to care for trauma patients. Critically injured trauma patients might be cared for by the ambulance emergency medical technicians, the rescue helicopter crew, the ED, the trauma OR, and the trauma ICU. The patient handoff between each of these departments is a potential source of error.

An example of a standardized patient data transfer sheet

FIGURE 5.4

"I M STABLE" TRANSFER NOTE		
I.D.–(Name, Age, DOB, MR#, Stat name, Sex)		
MOI–Mechanism of Injury/Chief complaint, Time of incident		
Status–VS, Neuro Status, Airway type	PTA	ED
Treatment–Meds, Procedures	PTA	ED
Allergies		
Background–PMH, Meds (home), Surgical history		
Last . . .–Meal, LMP		
Extras–Additional information/Injuries		

Report (Print name):

From _____ To _____

From _____ To _____

From _____ To _____

Fax numbers:
Trauma   3-1120

*Any entry should be documented with time or unit (LF, ED, etc.)
*Not part of medical record

Developed at Vanderbilt University Medical Center. Reprinted with permission.

The form is designed to flow though this maze of care with the patient, each caregiver adding to the information flow. No longer must each person along the way rewrite the data that were passed to him or her. The form can be copied and faxed to units that are expecting the patient, eliminating hurried and stressful phone calls between staff. For critically injured patients whose lives depend on getting to the OR and ICU quickly, this form ensures they get there with all of the information that the staff needs to provide the best care. The form can be customized, or simplified to apply to other patient data transfers or to serve as a template for electronic data transfer.

PACU Patient Transfer Report Briefing Guide

Background: Long-haul commercial airline flights, such as the 15-hour segments from Tokyo to New York, normally carry two full flight crews. One crew rests while the other flies. Responsibility for the flight is transferred from one crew to the other mid-flight. This system ensures that passengers are never put at risk by overly fatigued crews.

When transferring control, the crews use a defined and specific briefing guide to ensure that nothing is missed. The end of the transfer brief signifies the formal transfer of control.

Healthcare organizations have a similar situation when patients are transferred from the OR to the post-anesthesia (PACU). Anesthesiologists and certified registered nurse anesthetists turn over the immediate care of the patient to nurses in the PACU. Many organizations have found this process to be rife with communication errors that can affect the care of the patient. In response, they have adopted a page from the airline experience and instituted a briefing guide to be followed by anesthesia staff when transferring the patient. Following the guide ensures that all critical information is always communicated in a consistent and standard format. By receiving the report in a standard format, the PACU nurse knows instantly whether critical data are missing.

An example of a PACU patient transfer report briefing guide can be seen in Figure 5.5.

Methodology: The briefing guide is usually prominently posted in the work space at the patient's bedside. This allows anesthesia instant and easy access to the guide. When anesthesia staff have completed all necessary paperwork and recording of vital signs, they will start the transfer process by asking the first question on the script, "Are you ready for the report?" This signifies to both parties that anesthesia staff are ready to

PACU Patient Transfer Report Briefing Guide

FIGURE 5.5

PACU Patient Transfer Report Briefing Guide

1. Are you ready for the Report?

2. Patient's Name.

3. Age.

4. Weight.

5. Significant Medical History.

6. Allergies.

7. Antibiotics.

8. Type of anesthesia or narcotics used.

9. Fluid totals & I/O

10. Blood loss.

11. Drains/chest tubes/packing.

12. Other significant information/Assessment.

13. Pain sheet signed?

14. What questions do you have?

Source: LifeWings Partners, LLC. Reprinted with permission.

conduct the report and avoids those situations where the PACU nurse is still assessing the patient and not ready to devote full attention to the information.

When the nurse responds, "Yes," he indicates he is ready to focus on and record the needed information. The format and sequence of the information can be arranged as desired but should follow the sequence of information that needs to be recorded by the PACU nurse.

Further, the system allows the basic patient information to be transferred quickly, helping care providers to focus on patient assessment and integrated information that is typically provided in a good handoff between two experienced healthcare professionals.

The briefing guide is completed with the final question, "What questions do you have?" Notice the form of the question assumes there will always be questions and more effectively opens the door for them. This form avoids the overused, "Do you have any questions?" That question has become commonplace and is often interpreted to mean, "The briefing is complete, and I am finished," thus closing the door on further questions.

Room Setup Checklist

Background: The "hybrid OR" at Vanderbilt is a new and exciting concept. Combining a cardiac surgery OR and a cath lab, it permits the surgeon to determine the patency of the blood vessels reconnected in coronary bypass surgery before the patient leaves the OR. Members of the OR and cath lab teams were cross-trained to be able to work in this room, and all the equipment from both OR and cath lab were combined in this one suite. Many pieces of heavy equipment had to be placed on rails crossing the ceiling, to be moved into place as needed. New personnel, newly combined teams, complex processes, and new equipment locations are the perfect set up for errors and patient-harming accidents. Therefore a number of new safety tools were put into place and practiced before cases began in this suite. The primary safety tool is the OR setup checklist, seen in Figure 5.6.

Methodology: A tools-development team was assembled to create the safety tool. The team identified a safety concern: It is easy to move the ceiling-mounted equipment incorrectly and injure an OR team member or the patient. Therefore, each piece of equipment needs a precise starting position for the beginning of each case. The checklist identifies those positions.

A checklist for setting up a Hybrid OR

FIGURE 5.6

Hybrid OR Room Set Up

Charge Nurse

CO_2 Gas Tank (2) . . . . Check
        Check that two (2) tanks are available in physician reading room and
        that both are indicating green.

Sterilizer . . . . Verify QC check

Circulator

Room. . . . . Damp Dust

Patient Identifiers . . . . .Clears Previous Pt Identifiers

Defibrillators . . . . Run Self Test
        Check to make sure that daily check has been accomplished. Make
        sure defibrillator is charged and that paddles are plugged into
        machine

Perfusion booms   . . . . Positioned

Big monitor . . . . Positioned
        Make sure that monitor is at foot of bed, but does not hang over
        the sterile field.

Lights . . . . Positioned
. . . . ON
        Align overhead lights with blue tape at their base. They are aligned
        properly when blue tape strips are in line.

Mini-Siemens Monitor . . . . Positioned

Camera (C-Arm) . . . . Controls Active
. . . . .Park Position
        Active controls and move camera in all ranges. Test emergency
        stops to make sure they work. Leave camera in fully retracted
        (park) position.

FIGURE 5.6

A checklist for setting up a Hybrid OR (cont.)

Table . . . . Controls active

Chargeable cart . . . . Check for Implants

Room Camera (Siemens). . . . . Pt Loaded

VPIMS. . . . . Pt Loaded

Witt . . . . ON
. . . . Pt Loaded

STORZ (displays) . . . . .Selected & Displayed

Warmer . . . . ON
. . . . .Blankets Warm
. . . . .Saline Warm

Bear Hugger . . . . ON

Witt Leads . . . . Place with Anesthesia

White Board . . . . Complete

Many complex mechanical and electronic systems are included and need to be quickly and properly set. Extremely competent, experienced nurses received extensive training on all of the equipment, but didn't want to have to rely totally on their memory for correct room setup every time. In response to this need, the tools development team identified all the important setup steps and listed each on the checklist. The setup checklist was tested and revised in proving runs. The team created an expanded version of the checklist to be used for training and reference.

The checklist was designed as a read-and-verify tool. A nurse sets up the room from memory, using standard flows and habit patterns. When complete, he uses the checklist to make sure nothing was missed, and all equipment is positioned, set up, and operating correctly. This process adds approximately 60 seconds to the setup time.

Read Files

Background: Major commercial airlines typically have between 4,000 and 10,000 pilots. These large pilot groups must react in a timely and consistent manner to changes in the operating environment. Disseminating critical changes to aircraft procedures, policies, or safety risks by word of mouth is inadequate. Someone always fails to get the word. Healthcare, like aviation, is faced with constantly evolving procedures and practices. In order to best spread the word, establishing a common read file is particularly efficient. The read file is the unit's collection of important policy and procedural updates and changes placed in a single location (usually a binder) for use by the entire team. For brevity, only important issues are presented in the read file, and team members are held accountable for reading and initialing each entry prior to beginning their shift.

This example is for a paper-based system. Many organizations have developed electronic systems that accomplish the same goal. Regardless of the level of technology used, the principle remains the same and can be used anywhere.

Methodology: The read file safety tool must first be established by unit or departmental policy. Second, the unit should identify the location where the read file will be maintained. A specific staff member or members must be assigned the responsibility for maintaining the read file. An important part of the policy establishing the read file will be policy language charging team leaders (e.g., charge nurses, etc.) with ensuring that all members of the team check the read file prior to each shift or work day. Third, it is crucial to keep nonessential material out of the read file. Avoid making entries about the date of the holiday party or the unit picnic, for example.

In daily use, members of the unit will do the following to use this safety tool effectively:

1. Unit leadership will determine whether new policies, procedures, safety warnings, or other operational matters need to be included in the read file. If so, the material will be written, assigned a tracking number, signed by the unit leadership, and placed in the read file (Figure 5.7).

2. Once the new information is placed in the read file, both the index page (Figure 5.8) and the signature page will be updated (Figure 5.9).

3. Upon arrival for their shift, each team member will locate the read file and check both the index page and the signature page to determine whether new information is available.

4. If the read file has a new submission, it will be indicated on the index page. The team member will turn to the new submission (Figure 5.7) and read it.

5. When finished reading the new material, the team member will turn to the signature page (Figure 5.9) and place his or her initials on the row next to his or her name and in the column under the tracking number of the new submission.

6. Early in the shift or work day, the team lead will check the read file signature page to ensure all assigned staff have read and initialed the new material.

To illustrate the use of the read file, let's look at an example from the cath lab. Nancy Berg is the unit secretary. She has been given the responsibility to check the read file daily to make sure everyone is current. A new submission, p. 05-05 (Figure 5.7), was entered into the read file last week. When Nancy checks the read file signature page (Figure 5.9), she sees that Jeff Cohen has not entered his initials next to his name under the 05-05 entry. Today is the first day Jeff has worked since last week. Nancy finds Jeff and alerts him that he needs to read and initial the read file. With this process, Nancy is sure everyone providing care today to a patient in the cath lab has the latest information.

Examples of Read File submissions

FIGURE 5.7

05 – 05

Date: 4/10/05

From: Dr. Roger Ball

Subj: Patient Verification

1. The charge nurse will check the patient record and verify the name of the patient by looking at the patient's arm banding and asking the patient for their name.

2. Any discrepancies between record, schedule and stated name will be firmly resolved prior to beginning any procedure.

3. If there were discrepancies during initial verification, they will be brought to the attention of the attending physician.

RB

05 – 04

Date: 3/15/05

From: Dr. Roger Ball

Subj: Code Procedures in the Cath Lab

1. If a patient codes in the Cath Lab, the following procedures will apply. All Cath Lab team members are responsible for adhering to this policy.

2. If any team member assesses the patient in critical myocardial distress, that team member will call a code.

3. Team members will attempt to stabilize the patient as able while awaiting the code team. One team member should ensure that an ECG is continuously connecting and recording.

RB

FIGURE 5.8

An example of a Read File index page

Cath Lab Read File Index		
ENTRY	**DATE**	**TOPIC**
05-01	1/1/05	Patients with active TB
05-02	2/15/05	Patient Consent
05-03	3/14/05	Controlled drugs
05-04	3/15/05	Code procedures in the Cath Lab
05-05	4/10/05	Patient verification
05-06		
05-07		
05-08		
05-09		
05-10		
05-11		
05-12		
05-13		
05-14		

Source: LifeWings Partners, LLC. Reprinted with permission.

An example of a Read File signature page

FIGURE 5.9

	05-01	05-02	05-03	05-04	05-05	05-06	05-07
Alexander	JA	JA	JA	JA	JA		
Berg	WB	WB	WB	WB	WB		
Cohen	JC	JC	JC	JC			
Cooper	ZC	ZC	ZC	ZC	ZC		
Crutcher	TC						
Ermini	SE	SE	SE	SE	SE		
Graves	EG	EG	EG	EG	EG		
Green	kG	kG	kG	kG			
Halton	HH	HH	HH	HH	HH		
Hampton	XH	XH	XH	XH	XH		
Kukowoki	VK	VK	VK	VK	VK		
McCord	Mac	Mac	Mac	Mac	Mac		
Miller	MM	MM	MM	MM	MM		
Pilon	BP	BP	BP	BP	BP		
Porter	wp	wp	wp	wp	wp		
Sirles	QS	QS	QS	QS	QS		
Swatman	FS	FS	FS	FS			
Weingartner	HBW	HBW	HBW	HBW	HBW		
Williford	www	www	www	www	www		

Source: LifeWings Partners, LLC. Reprinted with permission.

Checklist standardization

Well-executed checklists work. They produce real results—improved standardization, reductions in variability, fewer errors, and better outcomes. When organizational staff understand what a real read and verify checklist does for them and how easy they are to use, they will want one. This is both good news and bad. The good news is safety tools that work gain widespread acceptance and become the way to do business. The bad news is that creating checklists isn't as easy as it seems. When everyone tries to create checklists on his or her own, the benefits of standardization are lost. Utility and functionality suffer as well. Here is a story we hear at institutions pursuing CRM projects across several departments.

The boss says, "The cath lab has a great pre-procedure checklist. It is really improving their efficiency. We need one here." The result? Departments enter a headlong rush to create their own checklist and keep the boss happy. "After all, the cath lab did it, why can't we?" Soon, an organization can be awash with checklists and guides with a variety of forms, styles, and methods of use. Attempts at unit standardization can create institutional nonstandardization. To see an example of this, take a tour of your hospital and look at the instructional placards for bed operation attached to the hospital beds. No two are the same.

Airlines are faced with the same problem. The typical airline will have several types of aircraft, often manufactured by different builders, in operation. Each aircraft type will have its own operational checklists. As much as is possible, airlines seek to standardize the checklists between fleets. Wherever possible, common terminology, formats, and methods of use are employed even though aircraft types may be different. For example, all checklists will use the same font and font size. Even though they may contain different steps, all checklists will have similar formats. One checklist looks like another. Checklists in common usage across all fleets will even be given the same name in every airplane type. The before landing checklist in the Boeing 727 is similar in scope, length, size, format, and actions to the before landing checklist in the McDonnell Douglas MD-11 aircraft.

The reason for this effort at standardization is that pilots frequently train to operate different aircraft in the fleet. As they move from one aircraft type to the other, they use similar tools systems, with similar protocols for use and terminology. In short, while the actual steps on the each checklist may be different, the look, feel, style, and method of use are the same. Thus, fewer errors are made and flight operations are safer. Every time pilots learn to fly new aircraft in their system, they don't have to learn a new way of using the safety tools.

This concept also applies to healthcare institutions. To illustrate this point, look at the cath lab pre-procedure checklist (Figure 4.4) and the hybrid OR setup checklist (Figure 5.6). See the similarities in format, style, and design? Formatting is similar, with identical fonts and print sizes. Most important, the protocols for checklist use are similar. Any time a checklist or tool is needed and used, the healthcare professional using it should intuitively know how it works, because it works like every other tool designed in the facility. The result is fewer errors, less variability, and greater safety.

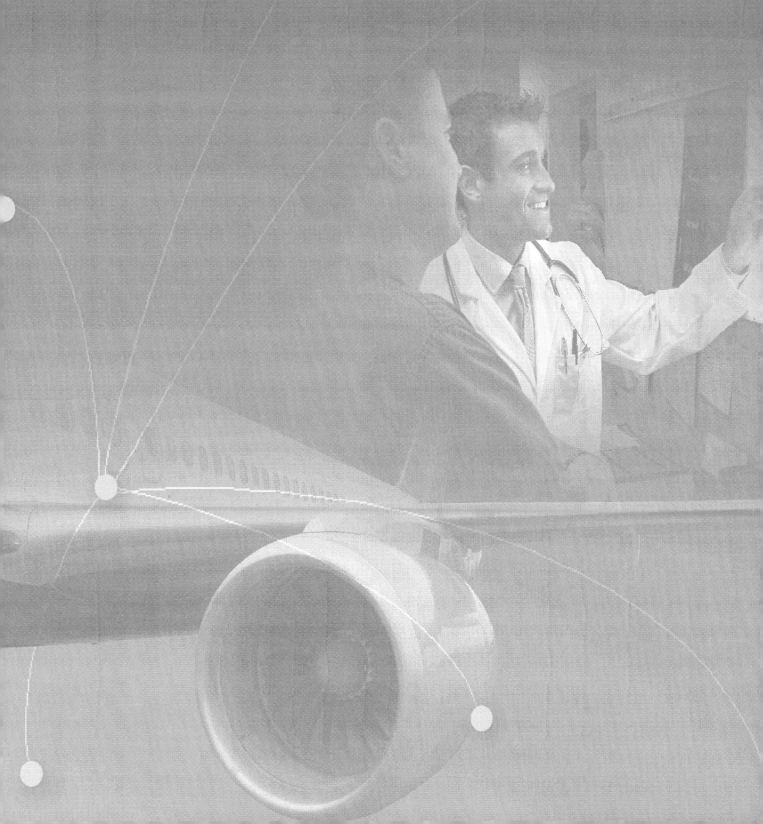

Chapter 6

OVERCOMING BARRIERS AND OBJECTIONS

Chapter 6

OVERCOMING BARRIERS AND OBJECTIONS

Despite following a successful flight plan and ensuring that the critical components of an effective CRM program are in place, organizational inertia may set in. In the end, a successful CRM project changes the way healthcare does business. Change is always hard. People resist it. Healthcare professionals are no different, and the CRM project leader should expect resistance. Be prepared to meet it head on.

One surefire preparation method is to make a list of the expected arguments against proceeding with the program. Most points of resistance are revealed in the loaded questions asked by those who will be affected by the project. The questions are loaded in the sense that each has an underlying message. The key to answering the question lies in understanding the hidden message and responding to it.

These questions are not unique; they've been asked everywhere in every institution that has embarked upon a CRM project. Here's a list of the some of the most common:

- Isn't this just airline stuff? How can you prove it works in healthcare?

- We'll be liable if teamwork becomes the accepted standard of care.

- I don't have time for all the training. I can give you one hour, but not eight. Can't you shorten the requirement?

- We're different here. Although I can see why it might work at General Hospital, what makes you think it will work here?

- With all the financial pressure this organization is under, why are we spending money on this?

Treat these questions like "hot grounders," the sharply hit ground balls a third baseman must field. He is able to make a clean play on the ball because of many hours practicing his response to sizzling grounders. Like the third baseman, you must prepare for the hot-grounder questions by knowing what questions will likely be asked, understanding the underlying message, and planning the best response to the message in the subtext. Once prepared, practice the responses until they become second nature. Then, you'll field them as cleanly as a major-league third baseman.

For example, let's examine this hot-grounder question:

"We'll be liable if teamwork becomes the accepted standard of care."

The underlying message is this: "We'll be sued. We fear change. We'll all be expected to do this. We don't want a new standard to operate by. This makes it harder on us."

Now prepare your response. Think about how to best respond to the underlying message. Ask several coworkers for their ideas. Collaborate and develop the best answer—one that makes sense for your organization. Whatever the prepared answer, always validate the questioner's concern by starting your response with this preface, "Yes, many others have had the same concern . . ."

Now train everyone involved in project leadership to respond similarly to this question. Ensure that all program leaders can and will respond on message. When complete, your response might sound something like this:

"Yes, many others have had the same question and concerns. And this program is the right thing to do for the safety of our patients. When it does become our standard of care, there will be fewer errors that harm patients, and therefore less risk of a lawsuit."

Repeatedly practice this response, out loud, until it becomes second nature. Follow the same process for each commonly asked question and for any other common lines of resistance developed in your organization.

Now try some of these on your own. We'll give you the question or comment. In the space provided, write down what you believe to be the underlying message in the question. Don't rush; rather, think about each question for a moment and reflect on the real concern embedded in it.

Next, formulate an answer that responds to the unspoken concern or message in the question. Write your answer in the space provided.

At the end of this chapter, we have included a table of common questions and the responses we have found to be most effective. However, we urge you not to skip this important exercise or to flip ahead to the table. One thing we know for sure in our work with organizations desiring to pursue CRM programs— you will encounter resistance. But this is not an barrier that is impossible to overcome. Preparation and practice will provide the tools you need to move forward.

1. *There can only be one person in charge. This program will undermine my authority.*

Underlying message/unspoken concern: _____

_____

_____

Response: _____

_____

_____

2. *What if I do "speak up" and get yelled at, or worse . . . ?*

Underlying message/unspoken concern: _____

_____

_____

Response: _____

_____

_____

3. *This takes time, and time is money; I'm already overbooked; etc.*

Underlying message/unspoken concern: _____

_____

_____

Response: _____

_____

_____

4. *CRM is okay, but not in an emergency.*

Underlying message/unspoken concern: _____

_____

_____

Response: _____

_____

_____

5. *I just don't buy CRM, and I'm not going to do it.*

Underlying message/unspoken concern: _____

_____

_____

Response: _____

_____

_____

Now, compare your answers with the information contained in Figure 6.1. We've put together what we learned in working with organizations to overcome resistance to their CRM programs. Use what works for your specific circumstance and discard the rest.

Refine your answers and practice, practice, practice.

	Effective responses to typical objections to CRM raised by 'slow adopters'
FIGURE 6.1	
Loss of authority	This is probably the most common concern of physicians. It is not always directly articulated, but rather suggested by such phrases as "There can only be one person in charge," or "There can be only one captain of the ship!'" In fact, the goal of CRM is to use all available resources, i.e. the entire team, to make better decisions. Making better decisions enhances the leader's authority. Remember, CRM was developed for very hierarchical airline and military aircraft crews. The "captain's" authority in those organizations was enhanced, not diminished.
What if I do speak up and get yelled at, or worse … ?	This is the most common concern expressed by staff members. The institution is giving CRM training to all members of the healthcare team. The leader of the team has made a commitment to listen if the team members commit to speaking up when there is a patient safety or other important issue identified. The benefit of having everyone looking out for the patient and the team is self-evident. The institution must also have made clear to everyone that CRM principles and practices are encouraged and "put-downs" are unacceptable. Finally, the individual has a choice: He or she can speak up when patient safety is at stake, or remain silent. It's our obligation as healthcare professionals to intervene when patient safety is at stake. Isn't it better to get "yelled at" than spend the rest of your life feeling guilty because silence led to patient injury? The institution must make absolutely clear that ignoring or becoming hostile about questions is unacceptable behavior, and be prepared to deal with it when it inevitably occurs. Everyone will be watching, and failure to honor commitments in this area will greatly lessen the institution's CRM program effectiveness.

FIGURE 6.1	**Effective responses to typical objections to CRM raised by 'slow adopters' (cont.)**

This takes time and time is money; I'm already overbooked; etc.	Taking time to do something right saves time. How many times has a procedure or process been delayed because someone or something was missing? Taking a minute or so means having everyone ready, understanding what will be done, what each person needs to do and what equipment and supplies are needed. The actual time required to accomplish various CRM activities should be measured directly and fed back to the staff as they improve and become more efficient. Many institutions report increases in efficiency as a byproduct of becoming more safe.
CRM's okay, but not in an emergency.	Physicians tend to accept many of the CRM-based changes in normal circumstances, but believe there's no time for CRM in emergencies. Experience with aviation and other high-risk environments shows clearly that errors are most likely to occur in emergencies when departing from standardized, well-trained procedures. CRM is more important in unusual situations where adrenalin is flowing and error rates are always increased. This is best addressed by having well-trained physicians and staff use CRM in such settings and achieving higher adherence to accepted protocols (e.g. ACLS, ATLS guidelines, etc.).
I just don't buy CRM, and I'm not going to do it.	This is not a common response, but it is inevitable. It's happening right now with implementation of the JCAHO required **"time out"** (a classic CRM intervention) and the read back of verbal orders, etc. Discussion of specific objections to CRM is sometimes helpful. Frequently, CRM is "rolled out" pod by pod, unit by unit. People who refuse to participate in CRM can buy some time by ignoring the requirements or hoping no one is watching. But the institution has to decide, in advance, whether it's willing to accept refusal to participate. The "non-adopter" may be a major admitting physician, a senior charge nurse, etc. Is the institution ultimately ready to say the following? "Patient safety and CRM are not optional. We've listened to your concerns and have addressed as many as possible. At this point, we acknowledge your concerns and issues, but CRM is important to patient safety and the operation of this unit, and it is required." Hand washing, wearing a surgical mask that covers both nose and mouth, and doing the JCAHO **time out** were all debated and opposed initially, and all have become the standard of care.

	Effective responses to typical objections to CRM raised by 'slow adopters' (cont.)
FIGURE 6.1	

I've been doing the "Debrief" and nothing happens. It's a waste of time.	It's better not to debrief at all than to fail to address the issues identified in a debrief. If a drug is missing from the "crash cart" and is so identified, the code participants can reasonably expect that the drug will be there the next time. It should be likewise for a missing surgical instrument, a person missing from the preshift briefing, etc. A debrief that leads to improvement is enormously powerful. One that does not has a huge negative impact. Be prepared to respond and act on suggestions before soliciting them.
So I've been doing this CRM, and I can't tell any difference	Careful attention to outcomes measurements and feedback to the staff are crucial. CRM is about teamwork. The institution must provide the team members feedback about compliance and outcomes where compliance has been achieved. All members of the team, but especially leaders, must know the data well enough to quote them verbally when challenged. Instances or near misses and other "saves" related to CRM implementation should be widely disseminated whenever they occur. Preventing a wrong surgery or fixing a potentially serious medical problem before it occurs can be a powerful motivator for continuing a CRM program.

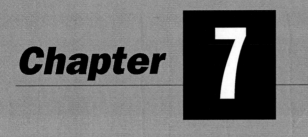

Chapter 7

CHOOSING THE RIGHT CRM PROGRAM FOR YOUR ORGANIZATION

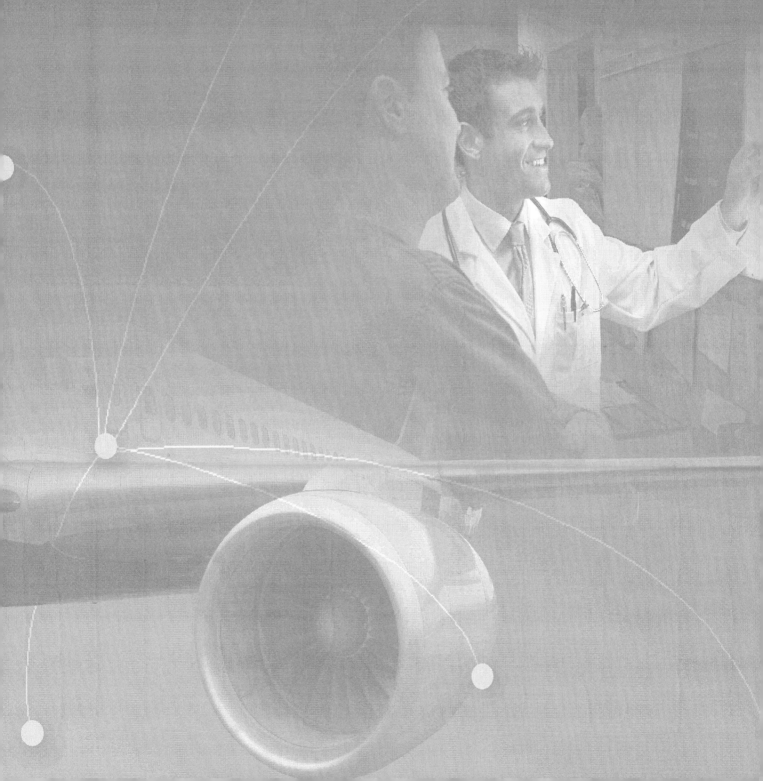

Chapter 7

CHOOSING THE RIGHT CRM PROGRAM FOR YOUR ORGANIZATION

What are the options for implementing a CRM program in your organization? CRM implementation in aviation has evolved over almost two decades and is highly standardized with surprisingly little variation among major airlines, airfreight companies, and the military. Although the blueprints are not identical, the similarities are far greater than the differences.

In contrast, healthcare's adoption of CRM is still in its infancy and shows great variability in approach and scope. Academic health centers, community hospitals, and hospital networks may approach CRM implementation based on their specific organizational characteristics, but there are some general principles that apply to all.

Experiences in both aviation and healthcare show clearly that the results achieved from CRM are highly dependent on the organization's leadership commitment, institutional capacity, and the level of resources applied. Because the CRM implementation options chosen by healthcare organizations will largely determine the results obtained, it's important to understand some of the different approaches taken and their risks and benefits.

The first steps in implementing a CRM program are to assess the organization's needs and then determine what resources are available to meet those needs. One resource already available to you is this manual. It provides a comprehensive blueprint with which to construct a successful program. Answer the following questions as you follow the blueprint:

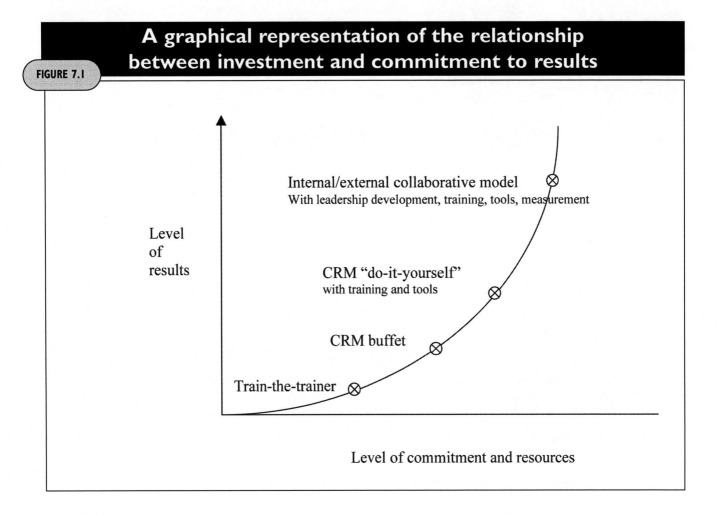

FIGURE 7.1

A graphical representation of the relationship between investment and commitment to results

Level of results

Internal/external collaborative model
With leadership development, training, tools, measurement

CRM "do-it-yourself"
with training and tools

CRM buffet

Train-the-trainer

Level of commitment and resources

1. What are your organization's needs? How much of the CRM program must you put in place to meet those needs?

2. How much of the effort needed to implement a CRM program can be accomplished by your internal resources? Does the organization have the time, personnel, and most important, capability to create the critical components of the program?

3. What financial resources are available to acquire the capabilities your organization does not possess?

Based on your responses to these questions, there are a number of options available. Each requires a different level of commitment and resources. Here are some of those options reviewed in light of the four critical components of a successful CRM program discussed in Chapter 4—Leadership, training, tools, and measurement.

Train–the-trainer CRM

This is the easiest and lowest-cost option. The institution decides it wants to implement a CRM program. Usually, there is a local champion who advocates a CRM program, frequently as a solution to a "problem area" where communication is particularly poor and/or some serious teamwork/communication-related patient mishap has recently occurred. Organizational commitment is not strong, but some funding is available, so the train-the-trainer approach is chosen. Following the principle of "See one, do one, teach one," an individual or a small team of nurses and physicians is sent to attend a CRM course. Such courses are available from a variety of sources, but most don't train attendees to be expert CRM instructors. If you choose the train-the-trainer option, pick a course that both trains CRM content and trains your team to be CRM trainers. This training should include courseware that is customized to address your institutional needs. Some people may not choose a true train-the-trainer course because CRM's common-sense, intuitive nature may suggest that it can be easily taught in a few hours. The thought is, "we just have to watch one, then we can teach one." Although the train-the-trainer approach seems attractive, it has several major limitations.

First, there is good evidence that merely sending employees to a class or two taught by your new trainers will not create lasting change in organizational behavior, process, or, most important outcomes. Some type of tools implementation is always required, so the focus should be on what specific skills or behaviors are being targeted. For example, some CRM skills are relatively stand-alone and can improve communication when properly taught. A CRM module on standardized communication could help produce a safety tool for standardized handoffs, and, if done properly, could also improve clinical efficiency and effectiveness.

The Joint Commission on Accreditation of Healthcare Organizations' preoperative time-out and read-back requirements are also prototypical CRM skills. These two concepts may be taught and implemented in a stand-alone program, especially given the fact that there's an external regulatory mandate to do so. Many of the other CRM skills and tools such as red flags, situational awareness, speaking up, briefings, and debriefings are much more linked and don't stand alone particularly well. In fact, increasing situational awareness without improving communication skills may unintentionally increase staff dissatisfaction without actually improving patient safety.

If the organization successfully implements a few basic CRM behaviors, it might provide the opportunity to go to the next step. However, the absence of leadership buy-in, a formal tools development program, and measurement of outcomes from initial efforts often makes taking the next steps difficult. In our experience, the type of results sought by most healthcare organizations come only with tools implementation. Without quantifiable results, leadership may conclude that CRM didn't work, when, in fact, it wasn't really implemented. Some organizations have had some benefit from the train-the-trainer approach, but not of the magnitude one would obtain from effort expended on a broader CRM program. Also, any observed change in the way healthcare providers work is based strictly on personal initiative, as no institutionwide structures were put into place to ensure that change is permanent. Leadership may find that some of the things that were fixed didn't stay fixed and will have to be fixed again in the future.

CRM buffet

Some organizations are able to provide significant resources for teaching and learning CRM but don't have sufficient commitment from clinical departments and their leaders for comprehensive CRM implementation. Staff, perhaps from the education/quality improvement department, can arrange CRM classes, visit institutions that have implemented CRM, and use consultants to develop internal expertise and the ability to develop and implement CRM tools. These skills and tools are then available internally on request. This approach allows units and staff to choose whichever CRM dishes they'd like without having to order a full meal. The buffet approach has the advantage of being relatively scalable and represents a pull, rather than push, change initiative. Full support from a given departmental chair or clinical director isn't necessary initially. Over time, the CRM training and tools produce pockets of real results and the benefits become better known. With persistent effort, a buffet CRM program can expand and become institutional and comprehensive, encompassing leadership, training, tools, and measurement.

CRM implementation by the buffet method is incremental and typically takes years, rather than months. It will require maintenance of significant internal expertise and/or long-term consulting arrangements. Outcomes are difficult to prove, and, in the long run, about the same amount of resources is consumed as would have been the case for a more focused, concentrated implementation program. Fortunately, it's relatively easy to transition from the buffet model to the next stage of CRM implementation.

Full do-it-yourself CRM

Larger hospitals, particularly academic medical centers and larger regional hospitals, may have substantial educational expertise and capability. These hospitals may decide to implement an extensive institutional CRM program largely on their own.

Before committing to a do-it-yourself program, leadership needs to ask several questions:

- Do we have a clinical unit where the probability of success is high?

- Do we have the resources to implement CRM successfully in that unit?

- While implementing CRM in that unit, can we develop an institutional infrastructure for implementing CRM institutionwide?

- Are we willing to commit those resources to implement CRM across the institution?

Leadership commitment and involvement are especially crucial to this approach because it is so resource-intensive compared with the other options. Dedicated personnel will have to be committed on a near-full-time basis. For some of these personnel, managing or working on this program will become their full-time jobs. For this approach to succeed organizations will need

- an institutional program manager

- someone to manage the skills training effort

- an institutional "trainer of trainers" to design and develop curriculum and train others at the unit level to provide it

- one or more trainers or unit-level educators

- someone to manage the effort of developing and implementing tools (in our experience, it is unlikely that the institutional trainer of trainers can do both courseware development and tools development)

- someone to manage the measurement program, perhaps from the institution's quality and improvement office

Prior to program start, all of the personnel identified will need extensive training in CRM, with a focus on the specific skills, behaviors, and tools discussed in previous chapters.

In this model, CRM really becomes a departmental program, with responsibility for development and implementation residing within the department's leadership. This guarantees local ownership of CRM and avoids any sense that CRM has been imposed or forced on the department externally. Experience with other improvement processes shows that local ownership is crucial for the long-term success and sustainability of the program.

The biggest challenge with the do-it-yourself approach is that the institutional and departmental personnel responsible for implementing CRM have never actually done CRM. Much of the work required to develop unit-specific CRM tools, practices, and procedures requires skills and knowledge not currently found in most healthcare organizations. This is especially true for developing useful, high-quality, standardized CRM tools such as read files, checklists, briefing and debriefing formats, etc. (see Chapter 5). The learning curve is steep, and it is easy to get off track, especially when developing and implementing CRM skills and tools into departmental workflows and processes. This is new ground for healthcare, and do-it-yourself efforts sometimes produce tools that aren't really effective CRM.

If available, templates and examples of proven healthcare CRM tools should be used until sufficient CRM material has been locally generated and refined.

The resulting CRM program will necessarily be iterative, so frequent, scheduled reviews with user feedback and objective measurement of compliance and outcomes should occur. What's working or not working and progress toward measurable outcomes must be assessed and appropriate course corrections made. Regular, direct observation will be necessary to know whether CRM is being practiced correctly. Computerized or written documentation of specific CRM activities (e.g., time out, invitation to speak up for potential patient safety issues, briefings, debriefing, etc.) are necessary, but they do not eliminate the need for direct observation to assess CRM compliance.

The institution's quality improvement or education department will ultimately need to create some "corporate" CRM expertise to ensure that information and skill transfer exist to roll CRM out to other departments. Development will be understandably slow with this approach. Other departments will see what is being implemented and will request similar opportunities. Although constricted resources (e.g., financial or, more likely, staff) may require that CRM implementation progress one department at a time, it's usually better to have a phased approach so preparatory work, involvement of unit leadership, classes, and tool development can begin somewhat in parallel within the institution. This avoids loss of momentum and makes efficient use of both internal and external resources.

The choice of this do-it-yourself model will be attractive to many institutions, but our experience is that it's complex and not as straightforward as it initially appears to be. The implementing unit has the authority and responsibility for the program as it develops it, and the unit's success or failure will determine whether subsequent CRM rollouts occur. Most large departments have multiple, competing demands for resources, of which CRM is only one. Local solutions may be favored over those with broader applicability, and the longer implementation takes, the greater the danger of both leadership and staff losing interest and commitment. Continuous, close collaboration between the unit and institutional leadership and both internal and external experts is crucial.

Network CRM implementation

Hospital systems usually have different needs and resources compared with single hospitals and can therefore approach CRM differently. Whether the hospital system employs its physicians has a major effect on how best to implement CRM. Support and consensus from nonemployed physician groups is much more difficult to obtain, and there is often no guarantee that having leadership on board will lead to widespread participation. Thus, finding champions for CRM and developing appropriate reward systems are important for a CRM program to succeed. Fortunately, many hospital networks have developed innovative approaches for winning affiliated physicians' support and can apply them to CRM.

Among hospital networks that employ their physicians, the Veteran's Administration (VA) probably has the most experience and success with CRM implementation in a hospital system. To do this, the VA's National Center for Patient Safety first created a dedicated, clinician-led team of physicians, nurses, and patient safety engineers. This team, working in collaboration with selected hospitals, and various CRM programs built curriculum materials and CRM tools suitable for implementation both inside and outside the VA. Their CRM course content generally is similar to the CRM curriculum described in Chapter 2.

When implementing CRM at a VA facility, the team first works with departmental leadership to identify needs and capabilities. They reach agreement in advance regarding which CRM tools will be provided and implemented. Compliance with JCAHO requirements determines some of the course content (i.e., time out, briefings, read back), while other high-utility topics of standardized communication, situational awareness, red flags, and speaking up are also included.

After completing the planning with the local hospital department's leadership, the national CRM team gives a one-day CRM course. All members of the department, including leadership, physicians, and staff are expected to attend the training course. Attendance is usually facilitated by closing the department for that day to complete the training. The last couple hours of the course are generally reserved for preselected team members to work on CRM solutions for specific unit needs.

Teaching by physicians and nurses trained in educational techniques and CRM content, specially created high-quality audiovisual materials that demonstrate CRM skills, and planned inputs from departmental leadership during the course create an effective learning experience. The course materials, including the videos, are used for additional locally managed teaching and review of CRM skills. The same team that taught the class also provides ongoing consultation and assistance with tool development and implementation.

Standardization, an important component of the VA's corporate culture, facilitates transfer of CRM tools across VA hospitals. Where physicians are not employees of the hospital or where there is great variability across hospitals within a single organization, a somewhat different approach is required, although many economies of scale are still possible.

In most hospital systems where the physicians are not employees, the first question to be answered is whether there is sufficient interest for a systemwide CRM implementation. If not, a program to create knowledge about and support for CRM as a specific improvement intervention should be developed. Once some support or at least interest in CRM exists, the same steps and requirements for implementing CRM in one hospital generally apply to an entire system. Most systems have some type of physicians' council and a nursing leadership organization. Support and consensus from these and other previously identified key leadership groups must be obtained. The same criteria for selecting a rollout unit in a single hospital can be used to choose the initial site or sites for CRM within a network. Once this is done, a collaborative CRM implementation model can be implemented.

Institutional internal/external collaborative model

With an institutional commitment, CRM implementation is more reliable and efficient and faster. Collaborative teams are composed of both departmental and institutional leadership and staff who will work extensively with external vendors, consultants, and colleagues from other institutions that have already implemented CRM. The external resources (e.g., consultants, vendors, and/or colleagues from other institutions) will not be able to implement a successful program in your organization on their own. It is the partnership between the internal and external resources that makes this approach work.

In selecting a specific unit or clinical area to begin your CRM program, leadership must assure that this is not seen as a "pilot project" but rather the first phase of a major institutional initiative. The area selected for initial implementation should have

- a strong interest in CRM
- committed leadership
- administrative stability that can accommodate major change
- unit capacity to support the internal work needed to develop unit-specific tools

This last point cannot be over emphasized. Lasting, measurable results are derived primarily from tools development and implementation. Although external resources can provide expert guidance for tools development and offer templates from which tools can be created, your staff must conduct most of the effort to implement the tools. This process requires close collaboration. The formula for success is internal sweat plus external knowledge and experience. Use this formula until you have developed the necessary internal level of knowledge and experience.

External consultants and experts will assist with or actually provide initial training of leadership, including the groups defined in Chapter 4. This accelerates initial learning so leaders can develop CRM implementation plans and tailor institutional policies to support the new CRM program and frees institutional resources for tool customization and measurement. This is consistent with the 80/20 principle (i.e., 80% of your result comes from 20% of your effort). Use your valuable internal resources on the part of the program that will produce the majority of the lasting results.

Trainers who have actively practiced CRM in aviation, healthcare, or both have high credibility with both physicians and staff. This credibility helps minimize initial resistance to CRM. A consistent, standardized curriculum closes gaps in learning and improves the quality and quantity of subsequent local input into tools development. Use of available tools and processes from the consultants and collaborating institutions also shortens implementation time. They should bring you tools with a proven track record at other healthcare organizations. Don't reinvent the wheel.

This external support and collaboration speeds the implementation of CRM. All four components of a successful CRM program can be accomplished sequentially in multiple units at the same time, rather than one unit at a time in sequence. For example, the cath lab can start its leadership training while the perioperative services unit, having already completed leadership training, begins its skills workshops while labor and delivery, having already completed its leadership training and skills workshops, begins tools development. Outsourcing of some aspects of the program such as training, at least initially, may provide flexibility in the timing of new unit starts, save time and staffing costs, and is usually cost-effective in the long run.

External consultants and colleagues from other healthcare institutions where CRM has been successfully implemented and CRM consultants are able to draw on their experience of working with these groups to continuously improve their models. Continued collaboration with healthcare organizations on tools development and measurement allows important methods for change to diffuse across institutions.

Over time, these organizations will develop important internal CRM expertise and minimize the problems associated with trial and error by each individual unit. An effective internal-external partnership will produce a repeatable, standardized program for implementing CRM programs in each department of the organization. Following this process produces a rapidly scalable CRM program: one unit or 20—it doesn't matter, just follow the standardized process.

The institutional implementation process will produce unit-specific tools that are standardized overall with respect to underlying CRM principles and key functions. For example, all procedural areas should follow the same basic format and methodology in developing

- a room set-up checklist

- a standardized process for transferring the patient from the holding room to the procedure/ operating suite

- the time-out briefing

- a debriefing format

When this standardized institutional implementation process is followed throughout the organization, efficiency improves and errors decrease because everyone knows what to expect and functions in a predictable, safe, effective way.

The same principles will apply when CRM is implemented outside procedural areas. Employees in nursing and intensive careunits will recognize a consistency in communication protocols and tools that tells them they are part of a team with standardized practices. CRM naturally moves organizations toward standardization, but only if their approach to CRM implementation itself is standardized. It is difficult to develop this level of consistency and standardization with previously described incremental methods of CRM implementation (i.e., train-the-trainer and buffet models).

The institutional internal-external collaborative model would be the best approach for most hospital systems. As with large hospitals and academic medical centers, initial partnering with CRM consultants and CRM experienced collaborating institutions allows transition to a more internally driven model as internal expertise is developed. If you choose a consultant to help you pursue this model, choose one who will help you develop this internal expertise as quickly as possible. A corporate CRM tools library should be established to shorten implementation time with subsequent hospitals.

Experience with CRM in both military and commercial aviation shows that significant decay in skills and practices will occur unless specific ongoing training and measurement of performance are conducted, so planning for ongoing and refresher training should be included in any systemwide CRM implementation. Success can be measured in improved outcomes, reduced medical errors and attendant malpractice costs, and by the extent to which other departments and hospitals within the organization begin requesting CRM implementation.

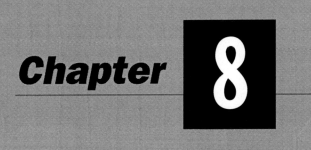

Chapter 8

PUTTING IT ALL TOGETHER: CRM IN ACTION

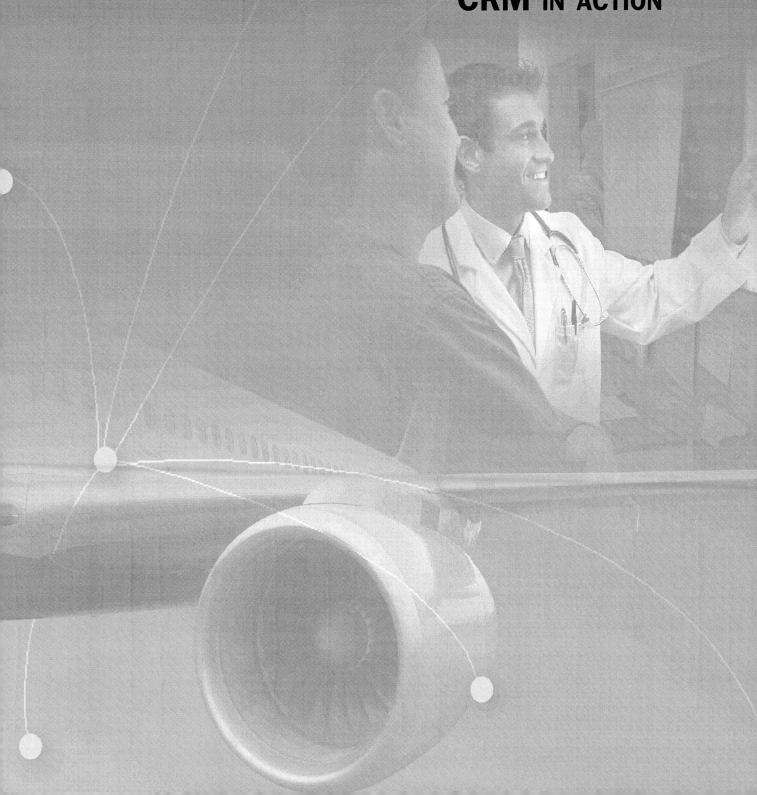

Chapter 8

Putting it all together: CRM in action

What could CRM do for your organization? Perhaps a story, based on two different scenarios from a real case study, can best demonstrate the lasting effect CRM can have on a healthcare organization better than any list of general benefits we might provide. The first scenario is what actually happened without a CRM program. The second represents what could have happened with an effective program in place. The story behind the scenarios is true. It actually happened in a hospital at which we later helped implement a CRM program.

Debbie, 34-year-old registered nurse, was admitted in active labor for the delivery of her fourth child at the same hospital where she worked. She had close friends on the staff in labor and delivery. She knew and trusted them. Her pregnancy up to this point had been completely normal.

After four hours of strong contractions, her obstetrician observed signs of fetal distress on the monitor. He conferred with Debbie and her husband, and together they made a decision to deliver the child via C-section. Her previous children were born vaginally, but because of a previous adverse reaction to an epidural anesthetic, the decision was made to use general anesthesia. The patient was prepped and taken to the delivery room at 2:45 p.m.

2:46 p.m. The anesthesia resident (AR) realized that the patient was her close friend. Worried for her friend, she expressed concern about the need for an emergency C-section to the circulating nurse (CN).

2:48 p.m.   The AR checked the pulse oximeter. She saw the alarm had been deactivated,   as often happened due to multiple false alarms.

2:50 p.m.   The patient was given a paralytic agent and IV sedation and was intubated by the AR. She checked the tube placement and administered general anesthesia.

2:52 p.m.   **AR (to the CN):** *"This looks right, doesn't it?"*
            CN: *"Do you have good breath sounds?"*
            AR: *"I'm checking that now."*

2:55 p.m.   **OB/GYN (to the AR):** *"Is the patient ready?"*
            AR: *"The general is onboard."*

            First incision occurs.

2:56 p.m.   The AR continues to check for breath sounds.
            CN: *"Did you ever get good breath sounds?"*
            AR: *"I think so, but I'm not comfortable with it, so I'm checking again."*
            CN: *"Are you sure it isn't in the esophagus?"*

            The AR does not respond.

2:59 p.m.   **Scrub nurse (to OB/GYN):** *"Does her blood look dark to you?"*
            OB/GYN: *"Yeah, it's darker than normal."*
            OB/GYN (to AR): *"Is everything okay? Her blood is very dark."*

3:00 p.m.   **CN (to AR):** *"Have you got it? Should I call for assistance?"*
            AR: *"No, I'm sure it's right. What did you say about her blood?"*
            CN: *"The doctor says it is very dark. What are her O_2 saturations?"*
            AR: *"Everything is fine; I haven't had any alarms."*

3:01 p.m.   The AR rechecks the pulse oximeter.

> **AR:** *"Oh my gosh, the alarm is off!"*

> The circulating nurse checks the pulse ox, sees a low reading
> and immediately calls for assistance.

3:06 p.m.   An attending anesthesiologist arrives, reintubates the patient, and
attempts to resuscitate the patient.

Miraculously, a healthy baby boy was delivered. The mother never woke up and was removed from life support the next day.

The family suffered a devastating, life-changing tragedy. The baby will never know his mother. The husband became a widower and single father in an instant. Angry and feeling completely betrayed by the people he knew and trusted, he ultimately filed a lawsuit. The hospital settled out of court for an enormous sum.

As well, this event had a devastating effect on the staff and the hospital. The AR was scarred for life and dropped out of medicine for almost a year. The rest of the team suffered with feelings of guilt and shame for months afterward. Their common refrain? "If only I had . . ." The entire department remained demoralized from guilt and self criticism.

It's difficult for this type of needless tragedy to happen in an organization that has implemented an effective CRM program. Here's why:

- Leadership has made safety a priority. Safety is listed as one of the corporate goals and all organizational leaders support patient safety by their actions. This support would be demonstrated in part by implementing a CRM program to help establish the culture of safety.

- Leadership's support of the culture of safety has made it clear to the team that they have the duty to speak freely about any concern affecting patient safety, with no fear whatsoever of repercussions or retaliation.

- Leadership has set clear expectations and accountabilities for the attendings. All attending anesthesiologists, as anesthesia team leaders, would have made it clear to all residents or nurses that they can get help when asked. When asked for any type of assistance, the anesthesia attendings would come immediately. This response would be consistent with the organization's written policies for such calls.

- All members of the team would have completed a comprehensive CRM course. During the course they would have demonstrated the ability to maintain situational awareness, recognize **red flags,** and communicate what they see. Because of that training and practice, they would be able to say the precise words, in the correct order, at the right time to convey the necessary message to prevent harm to the patient.

- It would be assumed that, even under the most carefully monitored circumstances, human error might occur. Therefore, every team member would cross check the performance of others and speak up when necessary.

- The AR's concern with the intubation and difficulty getting good breath sounds would have been recognized instantly as a **red flag** and brought to the attention of the rest of the team.

- During the pre-procedure brief, the obstetrician would discuss the intended actions. This briefing would include the entire team, including the anesthesiologist, and would be conducted using a checklist. The team lead would encourage team members to speak up if they saw anything affecting the safety of the patient.

- The pulse oximeter and any other needed safety equipment would be in place, tested in accordance with a checklist, and functioning before the procedure began. Testing would always include a functional check of any alarms.

- Had the hospital routinely conducted specific, objective, and non-emotional post-procedure debriefings, virtually all of the teamwork errors and shortcomings evident in this case would have been identified and addressed prior to the day this patient was harmed.

- Program measurement would have provided a clear picture of the level of compliance with the Pre-procedure Checklist and enabled the institution to reinforce the use of safety tools and teamwork behaviors. Furthermore, collecting data from the debrief process would have alerted the hospital to equipment problems with false alarms and they would have been previously addressed.

Thus, CRM improves patient safety by structuring the delivery of healthcare as a reliable process carried out by well-trained, effectively operating teams with defined objectives, responsibilities, and expectations of performance and outcome. Developments that fall outside of those expectations—whether the result of error, unexpected circumstances, or simple bad luck—are detected early with the use of teamwork and safety tools, communicated precisely, mitigated promptly, and discussed honestly and openly with the objective of improving the team's future performance.[1]

The first scenario of this case had a tragic outcome. As is the case in almost all medical errors leading to patient harm, there were multiple opportunities for simple interventions to have prevented the terrible outcome. Let's look at the same case again, but in a setting where leadership supported CRM, the staff had been trained in teamwork skills, safety tools had been implemented, and a robust system of measurement reinforced positive behaviors.

Debbie and her husband have just agreed with their obstetrician's recommendation that an emergency C-section is necessary.

The patient was prepped and brought to the delivery room at 2:45 p.m.

2:46 p.m. The AR realized that the patient was her close friend. Worried for her friend, she expressed concern about the need for an emergency C-section to the CN.

    CN: *"If something doesn't look right to you, say so and I'll call the attending immediately."*

2:48 p.m. The AR checked the pulse oximeter. She noted the alarm had been deactivated due to multiple false alarms. She immediately reactivated the alarms and checked them to make sure they worked.

2:50 p.m.   The obstetrician quickly called for the Pre-procedure Checklist as she gowned and gloved.

2:51 p.m.   The checklist was completed as the obstetrician said, *"If anyone sees anything that is unsafe or not in the best interest of the patient, I expect you to speak up."*

2:52 p.m.   The patient was given a paralytic agent and IV sedation and was intubated by the AR. She checked the tube placement and administered general anesthesia.

2:55 p.m.   **AR (to the CN):** *"This looks right, doesn't it?"*
     CN: *"Do you have good breath sounds?"*
     AR: *"I'm checking that now."*
     CN: *"If you are not sure, pull the tube and bag her. Let's call the attending while you do that."*
     AR: *"Right. Please call the attending for me."*
     CN (to the OB/GYN): *"Hold on Dr. Smith. The intubation doesn't look right and we're calling for the anesthesia attending now."*

2:56 p.m.   Just as the AR removes the tube, the pulse ox alarm sounds. The AR re-intubates the patient. The attending arrives. The attending checks for and hears good breath sounds.

2:57 p.m.   The attending tells Dr. Smith that everything is normal and to continue with the procedure.

3:07 p.m.   A healthy baby boy is delivered.

3:20 p.m.   As the obstetrician begins the skin closure, she begins her debrief. *"What did we do well on this case?"*

     CN: *"The time from the decision to do the C-section until we got the patient to the room was within our guidelines."*
     AR: *"We made sure the pulse ox alarms were functional."*
     OB: *"We caught the esophageal intubation and responded properly. Anything we could have done better?"*

Anesthesia attending: *"Always remember to cross-check breath sounds and what the pulse ox is telling you. If in doubt, extubate, bag the patient until the O_2 saturation is good, and then re-intubate."*

OB: *"Let's make a note that the pulse ox needs to be checked for false alarms. Thank you all for helping today. This is a happy day for Debbie and her husband; I know they will want you all to come by tomorrow morning to see their baby."*

The second version of this case study beautifully illustrates the point Dr. Don Berwick, one of the founders of the Institute for Healthcare Improvement, made as he initiated the "100,000 Lives" campaign. This initiative hopes to save those 100,000 lives that the 1999 IOM report says are lost every year in U.S. hospitals due to preventable errors. Here is what Dr. Berwick said:

> *The names of the patients whose lives we save can never be known. Our contribution will be what did not happen to them. And, though they are unknown, we will know that mothers and fathers are at graduations and weddings they would have missed, and that grandchildren will know grandparents they might never have known, and holidays will be taken, and work completed, and books read, and symphonies heard, and gardens tended that, without our work, would never have been.*

Toward this goal, we dedicate our work with CRM and wish you every success in your effort to implement CRM in your organization.

End note

1. Rosemary Gaffner, EdD, provided the basis of this description of CRM in her CME course "Reducing Medical Errors Through CRM" December 1, 2004.